HFMA Introductory Guide to NHS Foundation Trust Finance and Governance

Contents

Chapter 1	Acknowledgements	5
Chapter 2	Background to the Foundation Trust Movement	6
	2.1 What are FTs?	6
	2.2 Why were FTs introduced?	6
	2.3 How do FTs Differ from NHS Trusts?	6
	2.4 How do FTs fit Into the Wider NHS?	8
	2.5 Safeguarding NHS Patients' Interests	9
	2.6 Social Enterprises	10
Chapter 3	How FTs are Formed – the Application and Authorisation Process	11
	3.1 Introduction	11
	3.2 Development Phase	11
	3.3 Application to the Department of Health	11
	3.4 Assessment by Monitor	12
	3.5 Terms of Authorisation	12
	3.6 What the Future Holds for the Application Process	13
Chapter 4	Who is Responsible/Accountable for What?	14
	4.1 Introduction	14
	4.2 FT Members	14
	4.3 The Board of Governors	15
	4.4 The Board of Directors	16
	4.5 The Accounting Officer	18
	4.6 The Finance Director	19
	4.7 The Role of Committees	19
	4.8 The Board Secretary	22
Chapter 5	External Direction, Control and Regulation	24
	5.1 Introduction	24
	5.2 The Role of Monitor	24
	5.3 Monitor's Compliance Framework	25
	5.4 Monitor's Intervention Powers	29
	5.5 The Role of Other External Bodies	30
	5.6 External Audit	32
	5.7 What the Future Holds for Monitor	32

Chapter 6   Internal Control   34
              6.1   Introduction   34
              6.2   Foundation Trust Constitution – Standing Orders   34
              6.3   Delegated Powers/Decisions Reserved to the Board   34
              6.4   Financial Procedures   34
              6.5   Annual Governance Statement   35
              6.6   Internal Audit   35
              6.7   Risk Management   36
              6.8   Contracting   37
              6.9   Dispute Resolution   37
              6.10   Consultations   37
              6.11   Other Policies and Procedures   37

Chapter 7   Relationships with Other Organisations   38
              7.1   Department of Health   38
              7.2   Strategic Health Authorities   39
              7.3   Commissioners   39
              7.4   Specialist Commissioners   40
              7.5   Other NHS Providers   40
              7.6   Private Sector   40
              7.7   Banks   40
              7.8   Credit Rating Agencies   41
              7.9   Universities, Colleges and Further Education Establishments   41
              7.10   Local Authorities and Voluntary Organisations   41
              7.11   Overview and Scrutiny Committees (OSC)   41

Chapter 8   Revenue Funding   42
              8.1   Introduction   42
              8.2   NHS Income   42
              8.3   Non NHS Income   44
              8.4   Charitable Funds   46

Chapter 9   Capital Funding   49
              9.1   Introduction   49
              9.2   The Prudential Borrowing Code   49
              9.3   Affordability/Planning   51
              9.4   Public Dividend Capital Funding   55
              9.5   Sources of Borrowing   56
              9.6   Public Private Partnerships – the Private Finance Initiative   56

Chapter 10   Payment by Results   60
              10.1   What is Payment by Results?   60
              10.2   The Impact on FTs   60
              10.3   The Code of Conduct   60
              10.4   The Future of PbR   61

Chapter 11   Financial Planning, Accounting and Reporting   64
             11.1   The Annual Plan   64
             11.2   The Annual Accounts   66
             11.3   The Annual Report   68
             11.4   In Year Reporting and Monitoring – External   69
             11.5   In Year Reporting and Monitoring – Internal   70

Chapter 12   Treasury and Cash Flow Management   72
             12.1   Introduction   72
             12.2   What is Treasury Management?   72
             12.3   Operating Cash Management   72
             12.4   Medium and Long Term Investments   74
             12.5   Business Cases   75
             12.6   Working Capital Facilities   75

Chapter 13   Direct Taxation   77
             13.1   Introduction   77
             13.2   Are Activities Taxable?   77
             13.3   Trading Subsidiary Companies   79
             13.4   Calculating the Profits of a Trade   79
             13.5   Calculation and Payment of Corporation Tax Liability 80

Chapter 14   Insurance   82
             14.1   Scope   82
             14.2   Property Expenses Scheme (PES)   82
             14.3   Liability to Third Party Scheme (LTPS)   83

Foreword

Over the years, the HFMA has produced a range of introductory guides to finance, accounting and governance issues affecting the NHS all of which are designed to provide reliable, accessible and – above all – easy-to-read reference sources for anyone who wants to get to grips with how the NHS is structured and funded.

The focus of this guide is the finance and governance regime affecting NHS foundation trusts. It has been developed by the HFMA's Foundation Trust Technical Issues Group and is aimed at anyone who wants to gain an overall understanding of the key financial issues that foundation trusts have to grapple with. It will be particularly useful to new board members, managers and anyone who wants to get a feel for what foundation trusts are and how they operate.

As with other HFMA introductory guides, this publication does not go into great detail or provide definitive advice – instead, it is structured in such a way that, if readers want to know more about any aspect they can follow the pointers given to further sources of information. In particular, it is important that readers of this guide use it in conjunction with the guidance that appears on Monitor's website – including key documents such as the Compliance Framework, Model Core Constitution, the Guide for Applicants, the Code of Governance and Risk Evaluation for Investment Decisions.

Members of our Foundation Trust Technical Issues Group have quality assured the guide but inevitably some references will date more quickly than others, particularly as we move towards the new structure of the NHS. There may also be issues that readers feel should be covered in more (or less) detail and we would welcome any comments or suggestions to publications@hfma.org.uk

We hope you find the guide helpful and informative.

Paul Briddock,
Chair,
HFMA Foundation Trust Technical Issues Group.

Chapter 1: Acknowledgments

The guide has been developed by the HFMA foundation trust faculty FT FINANCE, and specifically it's FT Technical Issues Group (TIG). For more details about the faculty please visit www.hfma.org.uk/faculties/ftfinance. The HFMA is grateful to all the members of this group and their employing organisations for their help and support. FT TIG members are:

Sarah Bence	HFMA
Stephen Bloomer	Royal Orthopaedic Hospital NHS Foundation Trust
Paul Briddock (chair)	Chesterfield Royal Hospital NHS Foundation Trust
Ian Child	Basildon and Thurrock University Hospitals NHS Foundation Trust
Steve Clarke	University Hospitals Birmingham NHS Foundation Trust
Kathryn Corben	Derby Hospitals NHS Foundation Trust
Lesley Evans	Birmingham Community Healthcare NHS Trust
Catherine Eyre	Guy's and St. Thomas' NHS Foundation Trust
Russell Favager	Wirral University Teaching Hospital NHS Foundation Trust
John Flint	Chesterfield Royal Hospital NHS Foundation Trust
Adrian Goodchild	Cambridge University Hospitals NHS Foundation Trust
John Graham	Royal Liverpool & Broadgreen University Hospitals NHS Trust
Graham Harrison	Berkshire Healthcare NHS Foundation Trust
Paul McAuliffe	Oxleas NHS Foundation Trust
Mary Pettman	Frimley Park Hospital NHS Foundation Trust
Graham Platt	Hampshire Partnership NHS Foundation Trust
Mark Stewart	South Devon Healthcare Foundation Trust
Mike Stewart	Royal Devon and Exeter NHS Foundation Trust
Lakshmy Subramanian	Northern Lincolnshire and Goole Hospitals NHS Foundation Trust
Ken Taylor	Royal Berkshire NHS Foundation Trust
Ray Thomas	Countess of Chester Hospital NHS Foundation Trust
Sheila Wilson	York Hospitals NHS Foundation Trust
Michael Wilkinson	Royal Bournemouth and Christchurch Hospitals NHS Foundation Trust

Thanks also go to Willis Limited, Insurance brokers for their contribution to the guide.

Editorial work was undertaken by Sarah Bence.

Chapter 2: Background to the Foundation Trust Movement

2.1 What are FTs?

NHS foundation trusts (FTs) were created as new legal entities in the form of 'public benefit corporations' by the Health and Social Care (Community Health and Standards) Act 2003 – now consolidated in the NHS Act 2006.

Public benefit corporations draw on the traditions of mutual organisations established under Industrial and Provident legislation. In practice, this means that each FT has a duty to consult and involve a board of governors (comprising patients, staff, members of the public and other key stakeholders) in the strategic planning of the organisation. Governors are in turn accountable to the members of the FT – who are the FTs patients, carers, staff and members of the public – who can stand for and vote in elections to the foundation trust board. This governance structure enables FTs to actively engage their stakeholders in shaping plans to make health services more responsive to the needs of individual patients and the communities in which they serve.

This form of public ownership and accountability is designed to strengthen connections between healthcare providers and their local communities and to ensure that services reflect more accurately the needs and expectations of the local population.

2.2 Why were FTs Introduced?

FTs were introduced to help implement the then government's 'NHS Plan', published on the 1 July 2000. This 10 year plan set out a vision for the NHS in England to become more responsive and effective; and deliver a higher quality of care and services resulting in improved outcomes for patients.

By creating a new form of NHS trust that had greater freedom from central government control and more extensive powers in determining what services should be provided to local populations, the government hoped to liberate the talents of frontline staff and improve services more quickly. Alongside FTs, the government placed a renewed emphasis on increasing frontline clinical and nursing staff, expanding the use of technology, developing and implementing new treatments and therapies and raising capacity. The original aim was that together these initiatives would combine to provide significantly enhanced access and reduced waiting times for primary, secondary and tertiary care.

Initially, applications for foundation status were restricted to a number of 'three-star' NHS trust organisations with the first wave of FTs being licensed in April 2004, by the newly formed independent regulator for foundation trusts known as Monitor. Up until 2010, existing NHS trusts were free to register an interest in becoming a foundation trust, working with their strategic health authority (SHA) to progress an application. Since 2010, it has been the government's target that the majority of the remaining NHS provider organisations will gain foundation trust status by April 2014.

2.3 How do FTs Differ from NHS Trusts?

The FT structure represents a model of local management where central government involvement is reduced. FTs are managed by boards of directors and governors and have new freedoms to develop their services in line with local priorities and raise funds directly from the private sector. In practice, this means that in many ways FTs operate on a similar basis to commercial organisations.

Foundation trusts possess three key characteristics that distinguish them from NHS trusts:

- freedom to decide locally how to meet their obligations – they can tailor their governance arrangements to the individual circumstances of their community and health economy, while reflecting the range of diverse relationships with patients, the local community and other stakeholders
- accountability to local people, who can become members and governors of the foundation trust
- authorisation and ongoing regulation by the independent regulator of foundation trusts – Monitor. Monitor also has powers to intervene if an FT fails to comply with its terms of authorisation (see section 5.4).

As far as the financial regime is concerned, the key financial requirement as set out under their terms of authorisation is that FTs must 'operate effectively, efficiently and economically and as a going concern' and 'comply with a range of operational and financial requirements'. One of the main financial targets is to remain solvent. Other key differences between FTs and NHS trusts are:

- there is no statutory duty to break-even. FTs can generate and retain a surplus each year for re-investment. FTs can also incur a deficit, although the regulatory framework requires FTs to demonstrate financial viability over the medium term
- there is no requirement to remain within an external financing limit (EFL) target, or remain within a capital resource limit (CRL). However, FTs are still required to pay a Public Dividend Capital (PDC) dividend to the government which is paid as a 3.5% return on the average of net relevant assets
- there is no access to 'brokerage' or one-off support from central government. FTs do not have access to financial support from the local SHA or the Department of Health (the Department) if they suffer financial hardship, liquidity or cash flow problems. FTs are monitored against their liquidity performance and must ensure that they have sufficient cash balances to meet current and future commitments. To support this, the majority of FTs have a committed working capital facility provided by a commercial bank
- FTs can retain the proceeds of sale of non-current assets which can be used for reinvestment in patient services
- FTs can decide locally the capital investment they need to improve their services and increase capacity. They are able to borrow from the open market, including commercial loans from banks and other private lending organisations, in order to support investment. Lending is subject to Monitor's guidance as set out in Risk Evaluation for Investment Decisions by NHS Foundation Trusts and is limited by the FT's Prudential Borrowing Limit (PBL) that Monitor has approved for the foundation trust. The PBL is part of the Prudential Borrowing Code for NHS Foundation Trusts, details of which can be seen in chapter 9.

The financial freedoms granted to FTs bring with them new responsibilities. In particular, new skills need to be developed within management teams, among finance professionals and board members. This should assist in the process of service development, business case evaluation, financial planning, treasury management and opportunities associated with joint ventures, mergers and acquisitions.

2.4 How do FTs fit Into the Wider NHS?

Despite being independent of central government control, FTs continue to remain part of the NHS with the primary purpose of providing NHS services to NHS patients according to NHS principles and standards. In particular, the public continues to receive healthcare according to core NHS principles – free care, based on need and not the ability to pay.

While FTs must operate to national healthcare standards, they are not 'performance managed' directly and are free to determine their own strategic direction subject to the rules and procedures set down by Monitor and its compliance regime (see chapter 5).

The diagram below shows how FTs relate to other parts of the current structure of the NHS:

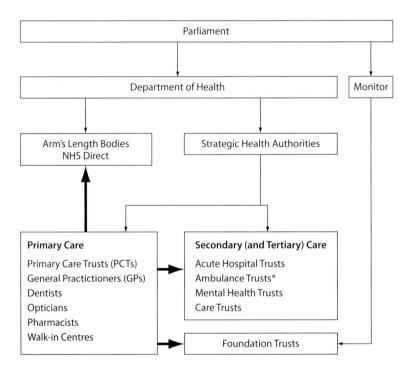

Key

→ Statutory relationship

➤ Planning, commissioning, agreeing care. Note that PCTs agree legally binding contracts with FTs and service level agreements (SLAs) with other NHS trusts.

*Ambulance trusts also work with NHS Direct and via the 999 system to respond to emergencies – this is regarded as part of primary care.

The diagram below shows what the NHS is likely to look like once the coalition government's proposals (as set out in the *Health and Social Care Bill 2011*) have been implemented:

Proposed NHS Structure

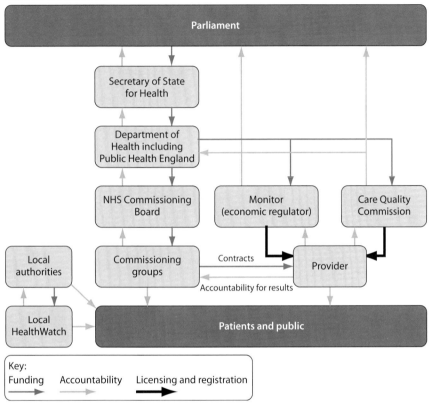

All NHS providers will be foundation trusts, jointly licensed by Monitor and the Care Quality Commission (CQC), providing health care services under contracts with clinical commissioning groups.

2.5 Safeguarding NHS Patients' Interests

To ensure that NHS patients do not lose out as a result of the introduction of FTs, there are statutory provisions set out in the NHS Act 2006, which place a 'lock' on the purpose of any FT. In particular 'mandatory goods and services' are specified in an FT's terms of authorisation – these are those goods and services that an FT must provide unless a variation is agreed first with commissioners and then with Monitor. Two other safeguards or restrictions stand out:

- 'protected assets': any proposed change in the use (including sale) of scheduled or protected non-current assets must be authorised by Monitor. Protected assets are identified at the time of application in terms of the protected services delivered from them. When authorising an FT, Monitor will take due regard of the protected assets for subsequent monitoring. Moreover, protected assets cannot be pledged as security for a loan

- private patient income cap: to ensure that the estate and future growth in services of an FT benefit NHS patients, the Act places a cap on the growth in private patient activity. Specifically, the Act makes it clear that the proportion of income from private activity as a proportion of total income must be no greater than it was for the predecessor NHS trust. In other words if private income was 3% of defined income in 2002/03 (in most circumstances the 'base financial year'), then it must not exceed 3% of defined income in 2003/04 and beyond. For mental health FTs, the cap on private income was amended by the Health Act 2009 so that it is currently the proportion of total income derived from such charges in 2002/03 (which for many trusts was 0%) or 1.5% if greater. The coalition government plans to remove the cap although FTs will be required to produce separate accounts for their NHS and private services.

2.6 Social Enterprises

Under the government's guidance within the 'Right to Provide for NHS staff', groups of staff or parts of organisations can form a staff-led enterprise where this is clinically appropriate. Open to all NHS organisations – not just foundation trusts, this model of service provision is based on a business case subject to approval by the current organisation's board. As foundation trusts are independent organisations, their boards are not obliged to support proposals for establishing staff-led social enterprises.

Chapter 3: How FTs are Formed – the Application and Authorisation Process

3.1 Introduction

At present, to qualify for authorisation to operate as an FT, applicants must meet stringent criteria set by the Department and pass Monitor's rigorous assessment process.

There are currently three stages in the application process for any aspiring FT. Initially the trust works with its SHA to prepare its application. It is the SHA's responsibility to make sure that the trust is ready and able to apply and become a foundation trust. The application must then be submitted to the Department's Applications Committee which recommends to the Secretary of State for Health whether or not the trust should proceed to be assessed by Monitor. If approved by the Secretary of State, the trust can apply to Monitor for authorisation as an FT.

3.2 Development Phase

Before an NHS trust can apply to the Department's Applications Committee and finally Monitor to become an FT it must first secure the support of its SHA. During this 'development phase' applicants must work with their SHA to:

- develop a five year strategic integrated business plan
- show strong leadership and commitment to modernising services
- demonstrate the involvement of staff and other local stakeholders for their vision for reform
- undertake a twelve week public consultation on their strategy and governance arrangements
- be subject to an 'historical' due diligence report by an accounting firm.

The integrated business plan must include:

- service development plans
- five year financial plans supported by activity, capital and workforce projections
- proposed governance arrangements
- an indication of how the FT's membership will help inform future plans and the direction of the FT
- a strategy for human resources including details of workforce requirements and involvement.

3.3 Application to the Department of Health

The second stage of the process involves the review of a trust's application by the Department's Applications Committee. It meets monthly to advise the Secretary of State as to which applicants should be recommended to proceed to the Monitor assessment phase. The Committee bases its recommendation on the evidence provided by the SHA but the final decision rests with the Secretary of State.

For more about the application process and the integrated business plan, guidance is available via the FT pages of the Department's web site and also on the Monitor website under guidance for applicants.[1]

3.4 Assessment by Monitor

Finally Monitor assesses the applicant for its financial standing, governance arrangements and management capabilities. Applicants meeting the required standards are authorised by Monitor, establishing them as an FT in the legal form of a public benefit corporation (as defined in the Act – see section 2.1).

In preparing for foundation status, trusts must demonstrate that they are legally constituted, well governed and financially viable. The main components of the constitution are:

- the eligibility criteria for membership and the designation of membership constituencies
- the composition and operating arrangements of the board of directors and the board of governors – including the role of the chair
- provisions for the conduct of governor elections
- circumstances when a governor or director may be disqualified or removed
- provisions for dealing with conflicts of interest
- details of the FT's 'registers' (for its members, governors and directors. For governors and directors the registers must include their interests)
- standing orders for both the board of governors and board of directors
- the appointment of the auditor
- the purpose of the audit committee
- the preparation and adoption of the annual financial plan and accounts.

3.5 Terms of Authorisation

The requirements placed on FTs are set out in their terms of authorisation prepared by Monitor.[2]

In particular, FTs are required by their authorisation to:

- put and keep in place, maintain and comply with arrangements for the purpose of improving the quality of healthcare provided by and for that trust
- deliver healthcare services to specified standards under agreed contracts with their commissioners

---

[1] For details of the FT application process and integrated business plan see the FT pages of the Department of Health's web site:
www.dh.gov.uk/PolicyAndGuidance/OrganisationPolicy/SecondaryCare/NHSFoundationTrust/fs/en
For details of the FT application process see the guide for applicants pages of the Monitor website:
www.monitor-nhsft.gov.uk/home/our-publications/guidance-applicants
[2] For more details see Monitor's guidance relating to terms of authorisation for NHS Foundation Trusts – available its web site: www.monitor-nhsft.gov.uk/publications.php

- maintain registration with the Care Quality Commission (CQC) and address conditions associated with registration
- operate effectively, efficiently and economically and as a going concern
- comply with healthcare targets and indicators
- govern themselves in accordance with best practice, maintaining the organisation's capacity to deliver mandatory services
- grow a representative membership
- cooperate with the CQC and a range of NHS and non-NHS bodies which may have a remit in relation to the provision of healthcare services
- disclose information to Monitor and third parties according to the detailed requirements set out in their authorisation
- deal openly and co-operatively with Monitor, including regarding potential or actual breaches of compliance with their authorisation or any serious reputational issues
- comply with statutory requirements, their authorisation, their constitution, their contracts with commissioners and guidance issued by Monitor
- follow the Principles and Rules of Cooperation and Competition and take such action as may be required by Monitor, advised by the Cooperation and Competition Panel, to address a breach of the Principles and Rules of Cooperation and Competition
- have regard to the NHS Constitution.

Monitor expects FTs to report any risks that could materially impact on compliance either as part of its normal reporting requirements or by exception.

In meeting the requirements of their authorisation, FTs must decide how best to organise and manage themselves so as to optimise the effectiveness, efficiency and economy with which they deliver services. They are managed by their board of directors who are accountable to members via the board of governors.

3.6 What the Future Holds for the Application Process

Under the coalition government's proposals NHS providers of healthcare will eventually all be foundation trusts – it will not be an option to remain as an NHS trust. Applicants will need to become foundation trusts as soon as it is clinically viable and will still need to pass Monitor's rigorous assessment process.

To support this strategy, the NHS Trust Development Authority will be established as a special health authority during 2012 with a view to taking over SHAs' current responsibilities for the foundation trust pipeline from 1 April 2013.

Chapter 4: Who is Responsible/Accountable for What?

4.1 Introduction

As we have emphasised, a significant feature of FTs is that they are released from direct Department control. Instead their functions are managed and executed through a board of directors and a board of governors.

4.2 FT Members

As mentioned in chapter 3, organisations preparing for foundation status must devise a membership strategy, which defines the membership community and appropriate constituencies from which governors are to be elected. This forms part of the FT's constitution.

FTs have a duty to engage with local communities and encourage local people to become members of the organisation. This duty is central to the mutual model on which the constitution of FTs is based (see section 2.1).

Legislation states that FTs must take steps to ensure that the membership is representative of the communities they serve. Eligibility criteria for membership vary between FTs depending on their local circumstances. However, the NHS Act 2006 requires FT members to fall into one of three constituencies as follows:

- a 'public' constituency – defined as 'individuals who live in any area specified in the constitution as the area for a public constituency'
- a 'staff' constituency – defined as 'individuals employed by the corporation [the FT] under a contract of employment and, if the constitution so provides, individuals who exercise functions for the purposes of the corporation otherwise than under a contract of employment with the corporation'
- a 'patient' constituency – for individuals who have attended any of the FT's hospitals as either a patient or carer of a patient within a period specified in the constitution.

Public and staff constituencies are mandatory but FTs are free to decide whether to have a separate constituency for patients/carers of patients.

All FTs are required to establish registers of members, directors and governors. These registers must, as a minimum, contain a list of names and, in the case of directors and governors, state their interests.

The board of directors should monitor how representative the FT's membership is and the level and effectiveness of member engagement. This information should then be used to review the FT's membership strategy.

'Model election rules' have been published by the Department to assist applicant trusts in drafting their constitution. The model rules include a proposed minimum timetable for the key stages in the election process, and the requirement that there must be independent scrutiny of the elections as overseen by a returning officer.[3]

4.3 The Board of Governors

The board of governors is made up of elected individuals from a wide stakeholder and community membership. When applying to be a member of the FT, an individual applicant can also confirm an interest in becoming a governor.

Legislation provides for each FT to decide on the size and shape of its board of governors in the light of their local circumstances, within certain minimum parameters set out in legislation:

- more than half of the members of the board of governors must be elected from the public and, where applicable, patient membership
- there must be at least three staff governors elected from the staff membership, or where there are classes within the staff constituency at least one governor from each class
- there must be at least one local authority governor, currently one PCT governor, and (where applicable) at least one university governor, all via nomination.

Monitor's Code of Governance also emphasises that 'the board of governors should not be so large as to be unwieldy'[4] and recommends that its role, structure, composition and procedures be reviewed regularly.

Governors are eligible to serve for a term of up to three years and to stand for re-election.

The board of governors represents the interests of the members and partner organisations in the local health economy in the governance of the FT. It may also be responsible for sharing information about key decisions with its membership community.

The chair of the FT is both the chair of the board of governors and the board of directors. This ensures that views from governors are considered by the directors and gives the chair a pivotal role in the organisation.

The board of governors is required to nominate a Lead Governor whose role is to chair the governors meetings when the FT chair is absent or unable to chair due to a conflict of interest.

The Lead Governor also has a direct line of communication with Monitor through which issues of concern can be discussed independently of the board. Such communication is not expected to be regular or routine, but is designed to enable urgent issues to be raised such as those concerning compliance with terms of authorisation, board leadership or where the process

---

[3] The model election rules can be found on Monitor's web site:
www.monitor-nhsft.gov.uk/home/search-results?search=election+rules&searchtype=all
[4] The NHS Foundation Trust Code of Governance, Monitor, 2010:
www.monitor-nhsft.gov.uk/publications.php

followed for board appointments or elections for governors has been questioned and communication through normal channels may not be appropriate.

A key role of the board of governors is to work with the board of directors to ensure that the FT acts in a way that is consistent with its terms of authorisation and to help set the strategic direction.

Monitor's Code of Governance gives more details about the role of governors and emphasises that they 'must act in the best interests of the FT and should adhere to its values and code of conduct'. The Code also states that 'the roles and responsibilities of the board of governors should be set out in a written document'. Specific responsibilities include:

- informing Monitor if the FT 'is at risk of breaching its terms of authorisation if these concerns cannot be resolved at local level'
- appointing, removing and deciding the terms of office of the chair and other non-executive directors
- approving the appointment of the chief executive
- agreeing with the audit committee the criteria for appointing, reappointing and removing external auditors
- considering the FT's annual report and accounts and its annual plan.

In October 2009, Monitor published separate guidance as to how governors may best deliver their duties entitled 'Your Statutory Duties: A Reference Guide for NHS Foundation Trust Governors' to provide them with more detailed guidance and additional support in carrying out the legal requirements associated with their role.

4.4 The Board of Directors

An FT's board of directors consists of executive directors (which must include the chief executive and finance director) and non-executive directors (NEDs). The chair of the board must be a NED. NEDs should have particular experience or skills that help the board function well. They are appointed by the board of governors based on recommendations made by a 'nominations committee' – see section 4.7.

The board of directors takes full responsibility for the governance of the FT and should present a balanced and understandable assessment of the FT's position and prospects. This responsibility extends to all public statements and reports to regulators and inspectors, as well as information presented under statutory requirements.

It is recommended that at least 50% of board members should be independent non-executive directors.

The board of directors has particular responsibility for:

- providing effective and proactive leadership of the FT within a framework of processes, procedures and controls which enable risk to be assessed and managed
- ensuring compliance with the FT's terms of authorisation, its constitution, mandatory guidance issued by Monitor, relevant statutory requirements and contractual obligations

- determining the FT's strategic aims, taking into consideration the views of the board of governors, ensuring that the necessary financial and human resources are in place to manage its performance and meet its objectives and then periodically review progress and management performance
- ensuring the quality and safety of healthcare services, education, training and research delivered by the FT and applying the principles and standards of clinical governance set out by the Department, the CQC, and other relevant NHS bodies
- ensuring that the FT exercises its functions effectively, efficiently and economically
- setting the FT's values and standards of conduct and ensuring that its obligations to its members, patients and other stakeholders are understood and met.

All directors have collective responsibility for every decision of the board of directors regardless of their individual skills or status and must take those decisions objectively. This does not revoke the particular responsibilities of the chief executive as the accounting officer (see section 4.5 below).

The role of NEDs is significantly different from their traditional role in NHS trusts. This is due in part to representation of local communities on the board of governors. As members of a unitary board, NEDs must take equal responsibility and accountability for the function and success of the business. They do have a particular duty to ensure appropriate challenge is made of the executive directors.

The board is required to nominate one of the NEDS to act as Senior Independent Director in consultation with the board of governors. The Senior Independent Director should be available to members and governors if they have concerns which contact through the normal channels has failed to resolve or would be inappropriate.

One particularly important duty placed on the board of directors and stated in Monitor's Code of Governance is that it 'must notify Monitor and the board of governors without delay and should consider whether it is in the public interest to bring to public attention all relevant information which is not public knowledge concerning a material change:

- in the NHS foundation trust's financial condition
- in the performance of its business; and/or
- in the NHS foundation trust's expectations as to its performance which, if made public, would be likely to lead to a substantial change to the financial wellbeing, healthcare delivery performance or reputation and standing of the NHS foundation trust.'

Monitor's Code of Governance also emphasises that 'the board of directors should not be so large as to be unwieldy'. For more details about this and the role of the board of directors refer to Monitor's Compliance Framework and the Code of Governance.[5]

---

[5] The NHS Foundation Trust Code of Governance, 2010 and the Compliance Framework, 2011/12: www.monitor-nhsft.gov.uk/publications.php

4.5 The Accounting Officer

The chief executive is the FT's 'Accounting Officer' – a statutory role originally set out in the Health and Social Care (Community Health and Standards) Act 2003.

The duties of FT Accounting Officers are listed in a memorandum issued by Monitor in April 2008.[6] This emphasises that 'Accounting Officers are responsible to Parliament for the resources under their control'. The memorandum also states that the accounting officer 'has responsibility for the overall organisation, management and staffing of the NHS FT and for its procedures in financial and other matters'. In particular he or she 'must ensure that:

- there is a high standard of financial management in the NHS FT as a whole
- financial systems and procedures promote the efficient and economical conduct of business and safeguard financial propriety and regularity throughout the whole NHS FT
- financial considerations are fully taken into account in decisions on NHS FT proposals.'

The memorandum also points out that the Accounting Officer's role is a 'personal responsibility for:

- the propriety and regularity of the public finances for which he or she is answerable
- the keeping of proper accounts
- prudent and economical administration
- the avoidance of waste and extravagance
- the efficient and effective use of all the resources in their charge.'

The role of the accounting officer (the chief executive) is a key element in corporate governance with a line of accountability stretching from the chief executive, via Monitor to Parliament.

Clearly the relationship between the chief executive and the board is an important one as he or she is responsible for 'ensuring that the board is empowered to govern the organisation and that the objectives it sets are accomplished through effective and properly controlled executive action'.

The NHS Appointments Commission has issued guidance that looks at the complexity of this relationship and although it does not apply directly to FTs it provides some useful pointers. In particular, the guidance summarises the respective responsibilities of the board and chief executive as follows:

'What the chief executive does for the board:

- helps create the vision
- provides information and expertise

---

[6] NHS Foundation Trust Accounting Officer Memorandum, Monitor, 2008:
www.monitor-nhsft.gov.uk/sites/default/files/publications/Accounting_Officer_Memorandum_April_2008.pdf

- provides operational leadership
- provides effective control systems
- delivers against operational objectives
- delivers the modernisation and change agenda.

What the board does for the chief executive:

- challenges and hones vision into high level strategic objectives
- supports the management of the organisation
- sets demanding but realisable operational objectives
- challenges and thereby reinforces the effectiveness of control systems
- supports the chief executive in making changes and taking risks by corporately agreeing plans and strategies and taking corporate responsibility for outcomes
- establishes a forward thinking, modernising and patient-focused culture for the organisation.'

4.6 The Finance Director

Finance directors are executive directors with a seat on the board. Their three key responsibilities as identified in the Finance Staff Development Board's 2006 guide to The Role of the Finance Director in a Patient-led NHS – a Guide for NHS Boards[7] are:

- to provide financial governance and assurance
- to provide business and commercial advice to the board
- corporate responsibilities as an executive director of the board.

Some FTs are now following a more commercial model with a chief finance officer focussed much more on finance and financing.

For more on the role of the finance director in the NHS and the skills, knowledge and qualities required to be effective see the HFMA publication 'The Role of the Finance Director' published in 2009.

4.7 The Role of Committees

Introduction

To help the board of governors and board of directors discharge their responsibilities effectively, FTs establish a range of committees. Some of these committees are mandatory – others are not. The key committees that FTs must – or are likely to – set up are discussed in turn below.

---

[7] Available via the library (documents) section of the FSD website: at:
www.fsdnetwork.com/documents/roleofdf.pdf

Audit committee

All FT boards must establish an audit committee. Monitor's Code of Governance states that this committee must be 'composed of non-executive directors which should include at least three independent non-executive directors'. At least one member of the committee must have 'recent and relevant financial experience'. Whether or not a NED is 'independent' is decided by the board of directors – Monitor's Code of Governance states that 'The board should determine whether the director is independent in character and judgement and whether there are any relationships or circumstances that are likely to affect, or could appear to affect, the director's judgement'.

The main role and responsibilities of the audit committee are similar to those of other NHS trusts, with the additional responsibility of making recommendations to the board of governors in relation to the appointment, re-appointment and removal of the external auditor and to approve the remuneration and terms of engagement of the external auditor.

The key guidance source for audit committees in the NHS is the Audit Committee Handbook[8] which states that 'The existence of an independent audit committee is a central means by which a board ensures effective internal control arrangements are in place. In addition, the audit committee provides a form of independent check on the executive arm of the board'. Although the Audit Committee Handbook does not apply directly to FTs the underlying principles are equally relevant. In particular, the Handbook's specimen terms of reference emphasise the audit committee's role in reviewing 'the establishment and maintenance of an effective system of integrated governance, risk management and internal control across the whole of the organisation's activities (both clinical and non-clinical), that supports the achievement of the organisation's objectives'.

Monitor's Code of Governance emphasises that there should be written terms of reference for the audit committee that include how it will:

- monitor the FT's financial statements and any announcements about its performance
- review internal financial controls and (if there is no dedicated risk committee) internal control and risk management systems
- monitor and review the effectiveness of the FT's internal audit function
- review and monitor the effectiveness of the external auditor
- develop and implement policy on using external auditors to supply non-audit services
- report to the board of governors any matters where action or improvement is needed and making recommendations as to the steps to be taken.

The audit committee should also review the FT's arrangements for 'whistle blowing' to ensure that they are both sufficient and accessible.

---

[8] NHS Audit Committee Handbook, 2011, HFMA: www.hfma.org.uk

Nominations committee

Monitor's Code of Governance emphasises the importance of there being a 'formal, rigorous and transparent procedure for the appointment or election of new members of the board of directors'. The Code goes on to say that a nominations committee should 'regularly review the structure, size and composition of the board of directors and make recommendations for changes where appropriate'. FTs may decide to have a single nominations committee that looks at both executive and non-executive directors or two separate committees. The committee should be chaired by an independent NED.

Remuneration committee

The remuneration committee is another mandatory committee that must be set up by (and report to) the board of directors. Its role is to set the remuneration levels for all executive directors and make recommendations in relation to the level of remuneration received by senior management (usually the first layer of managers below the board), including whether or not pay is linked to performance.

To ensure that people involved in the day-to-day running of the organisation do not make sensitive decisions in this area, the committee's membership is composed of NEDs and should include at least three independent NEDs.

See Monitor's Code of Governance for more details.[9]

Clinical governance committee

Although a clinical governance committee is not mandatory, NHS bodies have been advised in the past to establish one and it is good practice to do so. The key role of this committee is to review the organisation's systems to make sure that high quality healthcare is delivered. It is important to be clear about where responsibility for different aspects of clinical governance lies and to strike a sensible balance between issues that are considered by the board and those that fall within the remit of a dedicated committee. A clinical governance committee should report to the board of directors.

Risk management committee

Risk management committees are not mandatory. However, as FTs are required to have in place a comprehensive risk management strategy that identifies all potential risk areas, a dedicated committee is a good way of focusing efforts. In cases where risk management committees have been established for operational purposes (for example, to look at detailed health and safety monitoring) they may not be the appropriate vehicles for a more strategic approach.

In some organisations, risk management and clinical governance may be combined.

---

[9] The NHS Foundation Trust Code of Governance, Monitor, 2010:
www.monitor-nhsft.gov.uk/publications.php

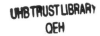

Whatever arrangement is in place locally the key requirement is that risks are identified, assessed and managed.

Investment committee

Although investment committees are not mandatory they are strongly recommended by Monitor as best practice 'if major investment is being proposed'.[10] Where they exist, Monitor identifies their key roles as being to:

- 'approve investment and borrowing strategy and policies
- approve performance benchmarks, review performance against the benchmarks
- ensure proper safeguards are in place for security of the NHS foundation trust's funds, monitor compliance with treasury policies and procedures
- approve proposals for acquisition and disposal of assets above a de minimis amount and approve external funding arrangements within their delegated authority.'

Monitor's guidance on operating cash[11] states that 'The investment committee should comprise executive and non-executive directors, with a majority of non-executive directors. It should be chaired by a non-executive director with relevant investment decision-making experience. It may therefore be a committee of the board, or the board itself in the case of smaller NHS foundation trusts.'

Other committees

FTs are free to establish other committees to suit their own circumstances – examples include finance and investment committees and finance and performance committees.

4.8 The Board Secretary

Some FTs have introduced a 'board secretary' role – this is akin to a company secretary in the private sector and is designed to ensure that board procedures, rules and regulations are followed. Although the board secretary is not a director he or she should have the equivalent status.

In its Code of Governance, Monitor states that 'the NHS foundation trust secretary has a significant role to play in the administration of corporate governance. In particular, the trust secretary would normally be expected to:

- ensure good information flows within the board and its committees and between senior management, non-executive directors and governors

---

[10] Risk Evaluation for Investment Decisions by NHS Foundation Trusts, Monitor, 2009: www.monitor-nhsft.gov.uk/publications.php
[11] Managing Operating Cash in NHS Foundation Trusts, Monitor, 2009: www.monitor-nhsft.gov.uk/publications.php

- ensure that board procedures of both the board of directors and the board of governors are complied with
- advise the board of directors and the board of governors (through the chairman) on all governance matters
- be available to give advice and support to individual directors, particularly in relation to the induction of new directors and assistance with professional development.'

Monitor goes on to say that FTs 'should give careful consideration to the appointment of a trust secretary in view of the clear benefits of the role'.

For more information refer to Monitor's Code of Governance.[12] The Institute of Chartered Secretaries and Administrators has developed a guidance note in relation to the roles and responsibilities of an FT Board Secretary – see: www.icsa.org.uk for more details.

---

[12] The NHS Foundation Trust Code of Governance, Monitor, 2010:
www.monitor-nhsft.gov.uk/publications.php

Chapter 5: External Direction, Control and Regulation

5.1 Introduction

There are a number of organisations that play a role in the regulation of FTs – this section looks at the key players.

5.2 The Role of Monitor

External monitoring and regulation of FTs is undertaken by Monitor in accordance with the FT's terms of authorisation. The authorisation sets out the basis for an FT's establishment and future operation.

Monitor is responsible for authorising, monitoring and regulating FTs and has established a 'risk-based Compliance Framework', together with other guidance, for the purpose of monitoring their performance (see 5.3 below).

Monitor's role is to assess risk to ensure compliance with all aspects of the authorisation and intervene if necessary where there is a significant breach of the terms of authorisation. To do this, Monitor relies primarily on the information it receives directly from FTs, but it also considers third party reports on a variety of specific issues, in particular those of other regulatory bodies.

The relationship of FTs with Monitor is based on effective self-governance and self-certification of compliance, with the board of directors taking primary responsibility for compliance with the authorisation. The chair has a key role in ensuring that the board of directors monitors the performance of the FT in an effective way and satisfies itself that effective action is taken to remedy problems as they arise.

FTs must initially report to Monitor annually (by way of an annual plan) and on a quarterly basis to ensure that they comply with their authorisation. However, as the compliance regime is risk-based, well-governed high-performing FTs are given space to exercise their freedoms and may, in time, be required to report less frequently, providing the FT has been authorised for at least two years and has been consistently in the lowest category of risk in each area. Where FTs are experiencing significant financial, service or governance problems, oversight is more intensive and monthly reporting may be required; intensity of monitoring will be guided by risk assessments.

Monitor has recognised the importance of effective governance in the success of every FT and has published a Code of Governance[13] to promote the key principles of good governance

---

[13] The NHS Foundation Trust Code of Governance, Monitor, 2010:
www.regulator-nhsft.gov.uk/publications.php

and how to apply them. The document is based closely on the UK Corporate Governance Code,[14] which is the nearest equivalent from the private sector.

5.3 Monitor's Compliance Framework

The Compliance Framework is designed to ensure that each NHS foundation trust remains compliant at all times with its authorisation.

Monitor has adopted a 'risk based' approach to regulation – this means that assessments of risk in a number of key areas are used to determine the level and depth of monitoring that an FT is subject to, such that intervention is only when necessary. The two key areas that Monitor focuses on are:

- finance and
- governance.

Monitor assesses the extent of the risk in each area by reviewing FTs' annual plans and in year monitoring submissions, the frequency and depth of which is determined by the FT's risk rating. Details of Monitor's Compliance Framework, its approach to risk ratings and FTs' current scores are available on its website. Monitor keeps the framework under regular review with a full update in March each year.

Finance risk rating

A financial scorecard is used to generate a finance risk rating (FRR) and this is split into four main criteria. For each criterion a score of 1 to 5 is awarded with 1 indicating a high risk of a significant breach of the authorisation and 5 a low risk with no financial regulatory concerns. The four areas are:

- achievement of plan
- underlying performance
- financial efficiency
- liquidity.

In practice, FTs are scored across five metrics which are compared to a grid of standard values, with financial efficiency being measured using two separate metrics. The five metrics are:

- achievement of plan – EBITDA (earnings before interest, taxes, depreciation and amortisation) achieved (% of plan)
- underlying performance – EBITDA margin (%)
- financial efficiency (1) – return on capital employed (%)
- financial efficiency (2) – income and expenditure surplus margin net of dividend (%)
- liquidity – liquidity ratio (days). Liquidity is defined as cash plus trade debtors (including accrued income) plus unused working capital facility (up to a maximum of 30 days) minus (trade creditors plus other creditors plus accruals) and is expressed in number of days operating expenses (excluding depreciation) that could be covered.

---

[14] The UK Corporate Governance Code, Financial Reporting Council, 2010: www.frc.org.uk

The box below explains why these metrics are used.

EBITDA and the risk rating metrics explained

EBITDA refers to earnings before interest, taxes, depreciation and amortisation. It is featured in two of the five metrics covering two financial criteria – achievement of plan and underlying performance.

Looking at EBITDA gives a different perspective on an FT's performance than simply looking at the bottom line. It is regarded as a good proxy for operating cash flow generated by the FT. As such it provides an indication of the FT's ability to reinvest in asset replacement and service innovation and to meet financing charges and dividends.

Unlike the overall income and expenditure surplus, it measures performance before depreciation, a non-cash accounting charge to reflect the consumption of capital, which can be influenced by matters such as asset life and other accounting treatments.

Achievement of plan: The achievement of plan criterion looks at actual EBITDA achieved as a percentage of the planned level of EBITDA. The annual risk rating is based on the achievement of plan in the previous year. All the other criteria in the annual rating (underlying performance, financial efficiency and liquidity) are forward looking.[*]

Underlying performance: The EBITDA margin measures EBITDA as a percentage of total income. It measures the extent to which operating expenses use up revenue.

Financial efficiency (return on capital employed): The return on capital employed is a measure of the organisation's surplus as a percentage of its asset base while taking account of everything it owes. The asset base takes account of property, plant and equipment as well as intangible assets such as software licences and includes money owed to the trust, stock held, cash and assets which can be quickly turned back into cash. The total amount owed by the organisation includes any finance leases including those relating to private finance schemes.

Financial efficiency (income and expenditure surplus margin net of dividend): The I&E surplus margin is a measure of how efficient the organisation is at turning income into overall surplus (after payment of dividend).

Liquidity: The liquidity ratio measures the organisation's ability to pay its short term bills. Monitor's definition, which importantly includes unused working capital facility funds as accessible cash, effectively measures how many days operating expenses the organisation could cover before running out of cash.

---

[*] In addition to the annual risk assessment, financial performance is also measured in-year using the same scorecard and rules. Unlike the annual plan assessment, which primarily takes a forward look, the in-year review focuses on actual performance in the most recent quarter and year-to-date.

Each FT is rated from 1 to 5 in each of these metrics and then using weightings, an overall aggregate FRR is produced. This is also a whole number from 1 to 5. A series of over-riding rules are then applied. For instance, an FT that has scored a 1 against one financial criterion, can only achieve a maximum overall risk rating of 2.

The weightings used to derive the aggregate FRR are:

- achievement of plan – 10%
- underlying performance – 25%
- financial efficiency – 40% (20% for each of the 2 metrics)
- liquidity – 25%.

As stated, one purpose of the FRR is to assist the regulator in determining the frequency with which he needs to monitor the organisation or intervene as appropriate. Another is to grant autonomy to high performing organisations in order that they may maximise the financial freedoms (including borrowing) and responsibilities available to FTs while at the same time ensuring proper risk management. For example, FTs will set their own level of capital expenditure and in so doing must decide on the best method of financing such expenditure. This can include:

- internal sources of cash such as depreciation, asset sales and accumulated income and expenditure surpluses
- Public Dividend Capital (in certain circumstances)
- borrowing through an NHS financing facility (see section 9.5)
- borrowing through an external lending facility such as a bank (subject to Monitor's prudential borrowing code (see section 9.2)
- the private finance initiative (see section 9.6).

Flexibility over capital expenditure is just one of the financial freedoms available to FTs – see section 2.3 for a reminder of the others.

Potential financial risk indicators

In 2010/11 Monitor introduced a range of additional financial risk indicators, used to highlight potential future material financial risk. These are not part of the formal regulating framework but all FTs must report and self-certify their performance against each indicator. The additional financial risk indicators are:

- unplanned decrease in EBITDA margin in two consecutive quarters
- quarterly self-certification by the trust that the financial risk rating (FRR) may be less than 3 in the next 12 months
- FRR of 2 for any one quarter
- working capital facility (WCF) used in the previous quarter
- debtors >90 days past due date account for more than 5% of total debtor balances
- creditors >90 days past due date account for more than 5% of total creditor balances
- two or more changes in finance director in a twelve-month period
- interim finance director in place over more than one quarter end

- quarter end cash balance <10 days of operating expenses or <£4m
- capital expenditure <75% of plan for the year to date.

Governance risk rating

The governance risk rating focuses on the degree to which FTs are complying with their terms of authorisation. Monitor looks at five criteria here:

- service performance
- third party views in relation to the CQC and the NHS Litigation Authority
- provision of mandatory services
- other certification failures where boards have failed to accurately self-certify and the failure is material
- other factors which can include failure to meet the statutory requirements of other bodies.

The level of governance risk is assessed using a graduated 'traffic light' approach where green indicates a low risk and red high. Monitor applies a scoring system to each level of risk as follows:

Green	A score from 0.0 to 0.9
Amber-green	A score from 1.0 to 1.9
Amber-red	A score from 2.0 to 3.9
Red	A score of 4.0 or more

Failure to deliver national requirements for example the clostridium difficile year on year reduction will adversely affect the governance risk rating. The weighting system also takes into consideration the need for all healthcare providers to comply with the registration requirements of the CQC (see section 5.5 below) and ongoing performance against those requirements. Subsequently, if the CQC raises 'major concerns' a score of 2.0 is automatically added to the FT's governance risk rating.

The provision of mandatory services

The governance rating incorporates the requirement to provide mandatory services. An FT is required to certify that it is able to continue to provide those services that are specified as being mandatory in its application for FT status and the terms of its authorisation. If an FT identifies a risk to this continued provision, the implications for overall governance will be considered by Monitor.

Service line reporting and management

Service line reporting (SLR) involves looking in detail at the revenue and costs of an FT's services in much the same way as a private sector company analyses its business units. In practice, this means that FTs look at profitability information by specialty. Monitor has issued guidance on SLR[15] which lists the characteristics of a typical service line as being:

---

[15] Service line management: an overview, Monitor, 2009: www.monitor-nhsft.gov.uk

- able to operate as an autonomous business unit
- having clear decision-making and accountability lines
- having clinicians in prominent leadership roles.

The information gleaned from SLR is used to 'manage' each service line and develop the FT's business plans with the FT overall effectively managed as 'a portfolio of autonomous and accountable business units'.

In its briefing 'Service line management: an overview',[16] Monitor states that SLM is 'an organisation structure and management framework within which clinicians and managers can plan service activities, set objectives and targets, monitor their services' financial and operational activity and manage performance'. The approach actively involves clinicians in business decisions. The briefing acknowledges that SLM is a developing area that will not achieve its full potential unless FTs have in place:

- well defined organisational structures and processes
- coherent operational strategies
- comprehensive annual planning processes
- information systems
- performance improvement policies.

SLR and SLM are regarded as best practice for FTs and Monitor's guidance is designed to help FTs develop their approaches.

Monitor's Compliance Framework for 2011/12[17] also requires that FTs with a financial risk rating of 1 or 2 in year report monthly analysis and EBITDA by service line for the previous year and the rest of the current year.

5.4 Monitor's Intervention Powers

Monitor has extensive powers to intervene in the event that an FT is failing to comply with its authorisation:

- the National Health Service Act 2006 (the Act) allows for Monitor to issue a section 52 notification for intervention, which empowers the regulator to remove the chair, chief executive, or an entire board of directors
- section 53 of the Act gives the regulator powers to ensure FTs 'take steps to obtain a moratorium' or a 'voluntary agreement' with creditors if it cannot pay them
- section 54 of the Act, allows Monitor to dissolve an FT in its entirety (subject to consultation). If an FT is dissolved, its assets can currently be transferred to another NHS organisation or the Secretary of State for Health
- the Health Act 2009 allows for Monitor to de-authorise an FT returning it to NHS trust status under the remit of the Secretary of State.

---

[16] Service line management: an overview, Monitor, 2009: www.monitor-nhsft.gov.uk
[17] Compliance Framework, Monitor, April 2011: www.monitor-nhsft.gov.uk

Monitor has significant powers of intervention if an FT is failing in its duties either from a clinical, governance or financial view point. These powers include requiring the board of governors or board of directors to take, or not take, specific actions. It could also involve the suspension of members of the board or governors and the appointment of interim directors.

For those FTs which may be or are in significant breach of authorisation on financial grounds, Monitor is likely to require the board to commission a report by independent advisers.

At present in the most severe situations, two courses of action are open to the regulator. The FT could be dissolved (subject to consultation) and all of its assets, staff and services transferred to another organisation. The 2006 Act provides for these measures to ensure the continuity and delivery of services to patients.

Alternatively under the existing legislation, the FT could be de-authorised and return to NHS trust status, following the issue of a de-authorisation notice by Monitor to the Secretary of State (section 52 of the 2009 Act). In these circumstances, Monitor must take into account:

- the health and safety of patients
- the quality of services provided
- the FT's financial position and
- the way the FT is being run.

Due to the significance of such action, prior to giving notice of de-authorisation to the Secretary of State, Monitor must consult with

- the Secretary of State
- the FT itself
- the appropriate strategic health authority
- relevant commissioners.

It is possible for the Secretary of State to initiate the process for de-authorisation by a formal request laid before Parliament containing an explanation underpinning the request. Monitor must then either issue a de-authorisation notice or publish its reasons for not doing so.

In the case of significant failure, any formal directions issued, or other actions taken under section 52 of The Act will be published in the public register maintained under section 39 of The Act.

5.5 The Role of Other External Bodies

The Care Quality Commission

The Care Quality Commission (CQC) is an independent body that operates at arm's length from the government and is responsible for regulating all providers of health and adult social care in England, be they NHS organisations, local authorities, private companies or voluntary organisations. It also aims to protect the rights of people detained under the Mental Health Act. It operates as a single regulatory body and supersedes the Healthcare Commission, the Commission for Social Care Inspection and the Mental Health Act Commission.

Following the introduction of the Health and Social Care Act 2008, the basis of the regulation is a comprehensive system of registration for all health and social care providers which came into effect on 1 April 2010. Services must meet essential standards of quality and safety and the operation of a single set of standards ensures that patients and members of the public know what to expect from all providers. The CQC monitors an organisation's compliance against the essential standards, with non-compliance resulting in enforcement action as is necessary and appropriate to the extent of the non-compliance.

FTs are required to register with the CQC as a provider of healthcare and comply with the requirements of their registration. A comprehensive list of the essential standards and details of the providers and activities covered by regulation is available on the CQC's website.[18]

Monitor and the CQC have a signed memorandum of understanding setting out the basis of their working relationship. They have undertaken to co-operate with each other and share information. In particular the CQC must keep Monitor informed of the provision of healthcare by NHS FTs and applicant trusts and any associated concerns it may have. Monitor undertakes to give the CQC any information it has about the provision of healthcare by an FT which either regulator considers would assist the CQC in the exercise of its functions. The memorandum is available on Monitor's website.[19]

In the proposed structure of the NHS (see diagram in chapter 2) providers of healthcare will need to be jointly licensed by Monitor and the CQC. Monitor and the CQC are to establish an integrated process for the licensing and registration of healthcare providers. Commissioners will only be able to place contracts for the provision of healthcare with those providers who are appropriately licensed.

National Clinical Assessment Service (NCAS)

The NCAS is a division of the National Patient Safety Agency. Its role is to 'promote patient safety by providing confidential advice and support to the NHS in situations where the performance of doctors and dentists is giving cause for concern'.[20]

In May 2006, Monitor and NCAS signed a memorandum of understanding which sets out the respective roles of the two organisations and how they will work together to avoid duplication. This memorandum is available on both NCAS's and Monitor's websites.

Other external bodies

There is a wide range of other organisations with an interest in health and with which FTs interact. These include:

---

[18] Care Quality Commission website: www.cqc.org.uk
[19] Memorandum of understanding between Monitor and the Care Quality Commission, 2011: http://www. monitor-nhsft.gov.uk/home/search-results?search=memorandum+of+understanding+DH&searchtype=all
[20] NCAS website: www.ncas.npsa.nhs.uk

- professional bodies on both the clinical and managerial side
- executive agencies, special health authorities and non departmental public bodies for example, the NHS Litigation Authority[21]
- local authorities – since January 2003, local authorities with social services responsibilities have been able to establish committees of councillors to provide overview and scrutiny of local NHS bodies by virtue of powers set out in section 38 of the Local Government Act 2000. The aim is to secure health improvement for local communities by encouraging authorities to look beyond their own service responsibilities to issues of wider concern to local people. This is achieved by giving democratically elected representatives the right to scrutinise how local health services are provided and developed for their constituents[22]
- representative bodies – for example, the British Medical Association (BMA), the NHS Confederation and UNISON
- think tanks and research organisations – such as the King's Fund
- the public – NHS organisations are required to engage with the public and conduct meaningful consultations.

5.6 External Audit

All FTs must have their annual report and accounts audited by independent external auditors who are appointed by an FT's board of governors. The audit will also report on consistency between the annual report and accounts and the FT consolidation schedules issued by Monitor. The external auditors also provide a value for money conclusion in relation to the FT's use of resources as well as auditing its quality accounts.

The audited annual accounts must be laid before Parliament. The chief executive, as Accounting Officer, may be required to appear before the Public Accounts Committee to answer questions.

The Audit Code for NHS Foundation Trusts, published by Monitor, prescribes the way in which external auditors carry out their functions.[23]

5.7 What the Future Holds for Monitor

Subject to the parliamentary approval of the *Health and Social Care Bill 2011*, the coalition government has proposed that Monitor will expand into a wider economic regulator for the health and social care sectors with an overarching duty to 'protect and promote patients' interests, by promoting value for money and quality in the provision of services'. To be able to fulfil this new role, Monitor will be responsible for licensing all providers of NHS-funded care in England, including existing foundation trusts, private and voluntary sector providers. This will allow Monitor to gather the information it needs to protect patients' interests, set prices and

---

[21] www.nhsla.com/home.htm
[22] To find out more about overview and scrutiny refer to the Department of Health's website (publications/ legislation) pages:
www.dh.gov.uk/en/Publicationsandstatistics/Publications/PublicationsLegislation/DH_4009607
Or visit the Local Government Association's web site: www.lga.gov.uk/home.asp
[23] Audit Code for NHS Foundation Trusts, Monitor: www.monitor-nhsft.gov.uk/publications.php

safeguard the continuity of services (see below). The licensing regime will replace the existing system for authorising foundation trusts and the issuing of terms of authorisation. If license conditions are breached, Monitor will be able to order the situation to be rectified and fine the provider if necessary. Monitor will levy fees on those it registers to support the cost of its licensing related activities but its other regulatory activities will be funded by the Treasury.

Monitor's three core functions will be:

- **setting and regulating prices for NHS-funded services**: the new regime will involve Monitor and the NHS Commissioning Board assuming joint responsibility for setting prices, with Monitor focusing on designing the pricing methodology and using it to set prices and the Commissioning Board developing the pricing structure. Clinical commissioning groups and providers will be consulted on the underlying methodology and will be able to raise objections
- **overseeing competition and integration**: Monitor will be able to apply competition law to prevent anti-competitive behaviour initially only for healthcare providers but eventually also for providers of adult social care
- **supporting the continuity of services**: Monitor will have a number of levers at its disposal to ensure essential services are maintained for the benefit of patients. These will include powers to protect assets, authorise special funding arrangements for essential services that would otherwise be unviable, levy providers for contributions to a risk pool and the ability to intervene in the event of failure if an organisation gets into difficulty (including powers to trigger a special administration regime).

Once the new regime is up and running, Monitor will no longer be responsible for the following activities:

- protecting taxpayers' investment in FTs – this will be assumed by a new banking function to be established by the Department. This unit will also be responsible for managing new public lending to FTs (a role currently carried out by the Foundation Trust Financing Facility)
- amendments to FT constitutions – although FTs will need to inform Monitor of any changes to their constitutions, FTs will in future confirm for themselves that they remain compatible with legislation
- accounting and reporting – the Secretary of State will take over the power to define accounting and reporting requirements for FTs
- information collection – the Department will collect information from FTs about their forecast spending.

Monitor will retain its regulator role in relation to the financial and governance performance of foundation trusts until 2016 when the emphasis will move towards governing bodies self-regulating their organisations.

Chapter 6: Internal Control

6.1 Introduction

FTs need to ensure that their system of internal control is operating in a way that is effective. This means having in place a range of processes and procedures which together ensure that the organisation is running smoothly and safely, keeping risks to a minimum.

6.2 Foundation Trust Constitution – Standing Orders

Standing Orders (SOs) translate an FT's statutory powers into a series of practical rules designed to protect the interests of both the organisation and its staff. In FTs, SOs are known as the core constitution. In many ways the constitution is similar to the memorandum and articles of association of a limited company or PLC. SOs for both the board of governors and board of directors are embedded in FTs' constitutions.

The majority of provisions set out within SOs relate to the business of the boards and structure of committees. This includes procedural issues such as:

- the composition of the boards and committees
- how meetings are run
- form, content and frequency of reports submitted to the boards
- what constitutes a quorum
- record of attendance
- voting procedures.

Other areas covered in SOs include:

- appointment of committees and sub-committees
- decisions reserved to the board (see below)
- standards of business conduct
- declarations of interest
- register of interests and hospitality
- duties and obligations of board members.

6.3 Delegated Powers/Decisions Reserved to the Board

A schedule of decisions reserved to the board and a scheme of delegation to other committees or officers is a detailed listing of what the board alone can decide upon and who the board empowers to take actions or make decisions on its behalf. FTs include these details within their SOs which form part of their constitution.

6.4 Financial Procedures

The rest of the NHS is required to have a set of standing financial instructions (SFIs) which cover financial aspects in more detail and set out detailed procedures and responsibilities. FTs are not required to have SFIs but do have written procedures that fulfil the same function and in reality many FTs have adapted the model Department SFIs to suit their own purpose.

6.5 Annual Governance Statement

FTs (along with all other NHS bodies) have to submit an annual governance statement (previously the Statement on Internal Control or SIC) as part of their annual financial statements. This requirement was set by the Treasury and the following disclosures have to be made:

- the scope of the accounting officer's responsibility
- the purpose of the system of internal control
- the organisation's capacity to handle risk
- a description of the risk and control framework including controls in place to meet obligations relating to defined benefit pension schemes, equality and diversity legislation, and CQC requirements
- a description of the key process used to ensure resources are used economically, efficiently and effectively
- a description of the steps which have been put in place to assure the board of directors in relation to quality reporting including the annual quality report
- confirmation that a review of effectiveness has been undertaken and that a plan is in place to address any weaknesses
- a description of the process for maintaining and reviewing the system of internal control and details of actions planned or taken to deal with any significant internal control issues.

The annual governance statement must be signed off by the chief executive, as the accounting officer, on behalf of the board of directors. The head of internal audit provides an annual opinion to the accounting officer and the audit committee on the adequacy and effectiveness of the risk management, control and governance processes to support the annual governance statement. This is an extremely important statement that covers the whole of an organisation – chief executives will be held to account if they sign a statement that subsequent events show they did not understand or take seriously.

Detailed guidance on the annual governance statement is available in Monitor's NHS Foundation Trust Annual Reporting Manual[24] and on the Treasury's web site.[25]

6.6 Internal Audit

All NHS bodies must have an internal audit service to provide an independent and objective opinion to the accounting officer, board of directors and audit committee on the extent to which risk management, control and governance arrangements support the aims of the organisation. Internal audit also provides an independent and objective consultancy service specifically to help line management improve the organisation's risk management, control and governance arrangements.

In practice this means that the role of internal audit includes:

---

[24] NHS Foundation Trust Annual Reporting Manual, Monitor, 2010/11:
www.monitor-nhsft.gov.uk/publications.php
[25] http://www.hm-treasury.gov.uk/d/2011_12_annex_2.pdf

- reviewing the adequacy and effectiveness of internal control
- assisting management in identifying problem or risky areas
- helping safeguard assets and resources
- highlighting areas of concern to the audit committee/board
- carrying out reviews/investigations
- liaising with external auditors/other regulators
- providing assurance to management/audit committee/board of directors that controls are operating effectively.

6.7 Risk Management

Risk management relates to being aware of potential problems, thinking through what effect they could have and planning ahead to manage risks. In this context it is important to recognise that no approach to managing risks can give an absolute guarantee that nothing will ever go wrong. It is also worth remembering that risk is about opportunities as well as threats. Good risk management encourages organisations to take well-managed risks that allow safe development, growth and change.

As well as underpinning an organisation's system of internal control, risk management plays a key role in the regimes of external regulators (see section 5).

The basics of risk management are simple – every organisation needs to:

- identify the strategic objectives and aims of the organisation
- identify existing and future risks that may affect those aims
- evaluate the potential impact
- identify ways of mitigating or reducing risks (for example, the Treasury suggests the four Ts – treat, transfer, tolerate or terminate[26])
- manage risks by putting in place controls and warning mechanisms
- continuously review the effectiveness of the approach and update as necessary.

Good risk management requires leadership and commitment from the top and ownership throughout the organisation. It is not about putting risks in a register and forgetting about them; rather it is about identifying and managing those risks, particularly those that present the biggest challenge in management terms.

The benefits of an effective approach to risk management include:

- reduction in risk exposure through more effective targeting of resources to address key risk areas
- improvements in economy, efficiency and effectiveness resulting from a reduction in the frequency and/or severity of incidents, complaints, claims, staff absence and other loss

---

[26] The Orange Book: Management of Risk – Principles and Concepts, HM Treasury, 2004. Available via the search function on the Treasury's website: www.hm-treasury.gov.uk/

- demonstrable compliance with applicable laws and regulations
- enhanced reputation and increased public confidence in the quality of services.

6.8 Contracting

The national contract model, first introduced with effect from April 2007, covers agreements between PCTs and all types of provider delivering NHS funded services including foundation trusts. It specifies detailed terms and conditions to be applied between PCTs and FTs and includes sections on pricing and payment, quality, service standards and targets, trust handling of risk, data flows, information reporting and demand management. It may also specify contracting arrangements where one PCT acts as a host for others in that SHA area. Copies are available on the Department's website[27] – see section 8 for more on revenue funding generally. These agreements are legally binding between the PCT and the FT.

6.9 Dispute Resolution

The national model contract contains clauses on the escalation of disputes to Monitor and SHAs as appropriate. Some FTs have chosen to use more independent arbitration routes in their contracts. This may include usage of the Centre for Effective Dispute Resolution (CEDR) model mediation procedures.[28] Should mediation fail, a referral would be made under the rules of the Chartered Institute of Arbitrators for final arbitration. Ultimately, court action may be necessary if disputes cannot be settled.

6.10 Consultations

As mentioned in section 5.5, overview and scrutiny committees set up by local authorities with social services responsibilities are empowered to scrutinise health services in their areas. Boards need to ensure that arrangements are in place to discharge these responsibilities.

Although the board of governors represents the interests of the FT's members and 'partner organisations' within the local health economy (see section 4.3), Monitor's Code of Governance makes clear that the board of directors is ultimately responsible for ensuring that there is satisfactory dialogue with its stakeholders and that members, patients, clients, staff and the local community are consulted and involved.

6.11 Other Policies and Procedures

For FTs to run smoothly, many more policies and procedures (both financial and non-financial) are required. These are usually pulled together in organisational policy and procedure manuals. These cover a wide variety of areas from banking procedures and use of credit/purchasing cards to freedom of information requirements, health and safety and equal opportunities policies.

---

[27] NHS contracts for 2011/2012 and guidance on the NHS standard contract 2011/2012 Model contract and model contract guidance, Department of Health, 2011: http://www.dh.gov.uk/en/Publicationsandstatistics/Publications/PublicationsPolicyAndGuidance/DH_124324
[28] For more details see CEDR's web site: www.cedr.co.uk

Chapter 7: Relationships with Other Organisations

7.1 Department of Health

FTs remain fully part of the NHS but are not subject to direction from the Secretary of State for Health. Instead, FTs establish stronger connections between themselves and their members and local communities.

An FT is not to be regarded as the service or agent of the Crown or enjoying any status, immunity or privileges of the Crown. The FT's property is not Crown property. This also means that FTs can enter into legally binding contracts with other NHS bodies and take action against them in the courts if necessary.

In August 2004, the Department and Monitor signed a memorandum of understanding which makes clear what each body's role is. This states that in relation to FTs and Monitor, the Department is responsible for:

- ensuring the policy and operational frameworks for the NHS are consistent with FTs operating effectively under their terms of authorisation issued by Monitor
- allocating resources to ensure that PCTs and other commissioners may purchase appropriate NHS healthcare provision to meet identified health needs
- ensuring that the Independent Regulator has the appropriate funding and access to any relevant Department information to discharge its statutory functions to the required standard.

The memorandum sets out the basis of the working relationship between the Department and Monitor and emphasises 'two over arching principles:

- the Department fully acknowledges the independence of the Independent Regulator and that FTs are not subject to direction by the Secretary of State
- the Independent Regulator acknowledges that the statutory responsibilities of the Department and its Ministers require them to continue to take an interest in how the Independent Regulator and FTs are contributing towards the satisfactory discharge of those statutory responsibilities so that the Department can ensure the continuing provision of comprehensive NHS services.'

The memorandum is available on the publications pages of Monitor's website.[29]

Under the government Alignment Project (Clear Line of Sight) Monitor's accounts will be consolidated with the Department for presentation to Parliament. This will mean that Monitor will need to guide FTs to the same accounting policies as the Department in order to allow

---

[29] Memorandum of Understanding between Monitor and the Department of Health, updated 2010: http://www.monitor-nhsft.gov.uk/home/about-monitor/how-we-do-it/working-partnership

simple consolidation. Monitor guides the accounting policies of FTs through the Annual Reporting Manual (ARM).

7.2 Strategic Health Authorities

FTs are set free from central government control and are no longer performance managed by SHAs. They are self-sustaining, self-governing, autonomous organisations that are free to determine their own future. The oversight role previously undertaken by SHAs is now performed by Monitor (see chapter 5). At present, the main remaining links with the SHA are in the areas of education and research and development income. An FT would normally have a legally binding contract with the SHA for the Multi Professional Education and Training Levy (MPET) – this is designed to fund education and workforce development in the NHS (see section 8.2). FTs may also continue to subscribe to the Finance Skills Development programme.

Following the proposed abolition of SHAs in April 2013 subject to the parliamentary approval of the *Health and Social Care Bill 2011,* the responsibility for education and training will transfer to a new special health authority, Health Education England.

7.3 Commissioners

FTs are accountable to commissioners for the delivery of NHS services through legally binding contracts.

The legally binding contract is usually based on a model contract issued by the Department, which is tailored to meet local circumstances, following legal advice taken by both parties. The main areas covered include:

- details of the commissioners who are party to the contract
- commencement and duration of the contract
- service specifications and targets
- activity, resources and payment terms
- information flows and the associated penalties if timetables are not met
- contract monitoring arrangements
- quality standards and the associated penalty regime for failure to meet the required quality standards
- variations to the contract
- dispute resolution procedure.

A new model contract is issued by the Department early each calendar year for the contracts relating to the coming financial year.

FTs need to obtain annual feedback and comment from commissioners on their plans for quality improvement, quality performance and measures to be used in quality reporting.

In addition to those commissioners with a legally binding contract with an FT, patients are treated from other areas, usually as emergencies, as 'non-contracted activity' (NCA). The commissioner responsible is billed accordingly in line with Payment by Results guidance where this is relevant (see chapter 10) or based on the price agreed locally with contract commissioners for non-PbR activity.[30]

With the proposed abolition of PCTs in April 2013 subject to the parliamentary approval of the *Health and Social Care Bill 2011*, the responsibility for commissioning the majority of healthcare will transfer to clinical commissioning groups. Led by GPs, clinical commissioning groups will work closely with local authorities to determine the services to be commissioned in line with local health and well-being strategies. They will also make use of a standard contract to ensure consistency and probity in the approach to commissioning.

7.4 Specialist Commissioners

An FT may have relationships with specialist commissioners for example, a cancer collaborative, with many such collaborative arrangements hosted by a single PCT. Under the proposed structure of the NHS, specialist services which are best commissioned at a national or regional level will be commissioned by the new NHS Commissioning Board from April 2013. Although the details are still to be confirmed, it is likely that the use of a standard contract will also apply here.

7.5 Other NHS Providers

FTs have legally binding contracts for the services they provide to and receive from other providers of NHS care.

7.6 Private Sector

FTs may have a relationship with private sector health providers (including treatment centres) in the form of contracts for providing NHS patients with care. In addition some FTs have private patient facilities via collaboration with a private health care provider. Again, contracts are in place for these services however, the amount of income which an FT can generate through the provision of services to private patients is currently limited by the Private Patient Income Cap (see section 8.3).

7.7 Banks

All FTs have relationships with the banking sector and hold commercial accounts as well as having a working capital facility (see section 12.6). Banks and other investment partners are used for the investment of surplus cash and FTs have a treasury management policy which specifies the maximum levels of investment and investment concentration allowed with each banking institution (see chapter 12). FTs are also able to operate government banking service accounts if they prefer.

---

[30] Further details can be found in DH Gateway reference 1160 'Who Pays? Establishing the Responsible Commissioner'.

7.8 Credit Rating Agencies

An FT is likely to use the services of credit rating agencies and its treasury management policy normally refers to levels of investments that are allowed depending on a bank/other investment partner credit rating. Most credit rating agencies provide free of charge details for the basic rating information, but other services are chargeable.

7.9 Universities, Colleges and Further Education Establishments

FTs will often work with local education institutions to further clinical training, in particular nurse training.

7.10 Local Authorities and Voluntary Organisations

Local authorities and voluntary organisations provide a considerable amount of social care. FTs work closely with these organisations to ensure the most appropriate treatment for patients and to assist in providing care for patients following an in-patient stay.

7.11 Overview and Scrutiny Committees (OSC)

FTs will often need to report proposed changes to services and the way they are to be delivered to OSCs. OSCs will also be asked to comment on the FTs quality accounts, quality performance and future quality plans.

Chapter 8: Revenue Funding

8.1 Introduction

Foundation trusts are entitled to certain financial freedoms however their clinical activities and related income sources are largely similar to NHS trusts. The majority of income is currently received from PCTs for clinical services provided to their patients. Most FTs (and non FTs) will also have a variety of other sources of income including clinical non NHS income, non clinical income and education and training funding.

Both FTs and other NHS trusts are required to use the NHS standard contract with their commissioners but for FTs this contract is legally binding. Contracts are currently issued for acute, community, ambulance, mental health and learning disability services.

The contracts contain details of how they are to operate including monitoring arrangements and procedures for the escalation of disputes. In recent years the contracts have increasingly focused on improving the quality of the care provided and now contain financial penalties for failure to meet key aspects of service quality. The contracts also contain a Commissioning for Quality and Innovation (CQUIN) incentive framework to reward the provider for the achievement of agreed goals on quality and innovation. In the past contracts were designed to operate for a three year period with the financial baseline and some of the schedules subject to annual renegotiation. However, from 2011/12 the contract has a standard duration of one year, the automatic expiry date being 31 March.

Where activity is not covered by a contract it is referred to as non-contracted activity (NCA). NCA activity is billed on a monthly basis in line with the reporting dates included within the standard NHS contract. In the main, NCA activity consists of non-elective work where patients are admitted to a hospital in an emergency.

8.2 NHS Income

Primary care trusts

At present, the majority of an FT's income comes from PCTs and – for acute FTs – the majority of this falls under the Payment by Results (PbR) regime.

Under PbR, FTs (and other trusts) are reimbursed according to a pre-set national price or tariff for each patient treated. PCTs pay for the treatment received by patients registered with a GP. This mandatory tariff is payable for day case, ordinary elective and non-elected admitted patient care, outpatient attendances, outpatient procedures and accident and emergency services.

PCTs and FTs agree a baseline level of activity within the contract and the cost of this is paid to the FT on a monthly basis. Under PbR money follows the patient so if activity exceeds the plan the FT 'over-performs' and charges the PCT for this excess 'over-performance'. If activity is less than plan the FT has under-performed and issues a credit note to the PCT.

For activity not covered by PbR, local prices are set through negotiation with the PCT. At present, this includes activity such as critical care, community midwifery and certain high cost drugs and procedures.

In addition to the national tariff 'High Quality Care for All'[31] set out a quality framework for the NHS and included a new payment regime – CQUIN which, as noted above, is reflected in the NHS standard contract. For 2011/12 the value of CQUIN payments is up to 1.5% of the actual outturn of the contract rising to 2.5% in 2012/13. Commissioners can withhold significant proportions of payments if providers fail to meet mutually agreed quality goals.

PbR does not yet apply in full to mental health trusts although a national currency (a unit by which activity can be measured) is now being used alongside local prices agreed within health economies. The currency unit is a 'care cluster' which focuses on the characteristics of a service user rather than the interventions a patient receives.

Local authorities

Many mental health FTs are party to agreements to provide mental health and social care services jointly with local authorities and PCTs. In some cases this takes place under legally binding agreements introduced under section 31 of the Health Act 1999. The aim of these agreements is 'to enable partners to join together to design and deliver services around the needs of users rather than worrying about the boundaries of their organisations'.[32]

In practice, this means that 'pooled budgets' exist where a local authority and an NHS body combine resources and jointly commission or manage an integrated service. The idea is that, once a pooled budget is introduced, the public will experience a seamless service with a single point of access for their health and social care needs.

Where a pooled budget exists, regulations require that the partners have written agreements which set out:

- the functions covered
- the aims agreed
- the funds that each partner will contribute
- which partner will act as the 'host' (that is, which organisation will manage the budget and take responsibility for the accounts and auditing).

Market forces factor

The market forces factor (MFF) is an adjustment to the national tariff set by the Department for each provider. This adjustment allows for the variation in cost base in different parts of the country.

---

[31] High Quality Care for All: NHS Next Stage Review Final Report. Lord Darzi. 2008.
[32] For more on section 31 agreements and Health Act 1999 partnership arrangements: HSC 2000/010: Implementation of Health Act Partnership Arrangements: Department of Health – Publications

The lowest cost base is deemed to be Cornwall Partnership NHS Trust which has an MFF of 1.00. Elsewhere in the country the MFF is above this – for example, most parts of London are between 1.20 and 1.25. The maximum of the range is 1.298 in 2011/12 relating to University College London Hospitals NHS Foundation Trust.

An FT (and non FT) will charge the national tariff to its PCTs plus the MFF for that activity. For example, if a provider with an MFF payment index of 1.2 does £100,000 of work for a PCT then the provider would bill the PCT £100,000 plus an additional £20,000 for the MFF making a total of £120,000. The same work done by a provider with an MFF of 1.0 would incur a charge of £100,000. Local prices are calculated by providers based upon their actual cost and so inherently include an MFF such that no further adjustment is necessary.

Until 2009/10, the MFF relating to activity covered by PbR was paid by the Department directly to providers as a separate sum rather than through an adjustment to the tariff. This was designed to avoid price based competition and discourage PCTs from directing patients to services provided by trusts in a lower MFF zone. However, from 2009/10 the MFF for PbR activity is included within each PCT's allocation from the Department.

Education and training

FTs receive education and training funding in the same way as other NHS trusts – the amounts involved can be significant at large teaching trusts. The sources of funding include:

- Non-medical Education and Training funding (NMET) – used to buy pre- and post-registration education and training for nurses, midwives, allied health professionals (AHPs) and other staff mainly at higher education institutions
- Medical and Dental Education Levy (MADEL) – used to pay for the postgraduate education and training of doctors and dentists
- Service Increment for Teaching (SIFT).

8.3 Non NHS Income

Private patients

Many FTs generate additional income through treating patients privately: either billing insurance companies or individuals direct. Since foundation trusts were established they have been restricted, under the terms of their authorisation, to the amount of private income they can earn by the 'Private Patient Income Cap'. This cap states the proportion of total patient related income that can be derived from private healthcare sources (see section 2.5). An FT is limited to the proportion of income generated by private charges of the preceding organisation in the 'base year' of 2002/03. FTs must publish their performance against the private patient income cap in their annual accounts. Any breach of the cap results in regulatory action by Monitor.

Under the coalition government's proposals, foundation trusts will have their private patient income cap removed but will need to produce separate accounts for NHS and private-funded services.

Ministry of Defence

A very few FTs (and other NHS trusts) have a Ministry of Defence (MOD) Hospital Unit within their trust. Within this partnership the FT will have two contracts with the MOD: one for training military medical personnel and one for treating military patients. Income relating to the treatment contract is paid directly to the trust by the MOD. The contract for treating military personnel mirrors the standard contract and uses PbR although it may contain the opportunity for additional 'premia' payments for treating military personnel in faster time frames than would normally apply to civilian NHS patients.

Research and development

FTs can receive funding for research and development in the same way as other NHS trusts – see the Department's website for details.[33]

Overseas visitors

FTs (and other NHS trusts) charge for overseas visitors in one of two ways:

- 'charge exempt' – mainly people from countries where a reciprocal agreement exists with the UK (for example, the European Economic Area or EEA). There are also certain diseases and some other exemptions that fall under this heading. The costs are billed to the host PCT using the standard tariff
- 'other' – all other foreign nationals are chargeable for their treatment apart from that received within accident and emergency and in the treatment of certain diseases (as in the case of charge exempt patients).

Catering and car parks

Many FTs (and other trusts) charge staff and visitors for parking, canteens, sandwich shops, cafes etc.

Injury costs recovery

The Injury Costs Recovery (ICR) scheme came into effect in January 2007 and replaced the Road Traffic Act (RTA) scheme. The ICR scheme expands the range of cases where the NHS can reclaim the cost of treating injured patients to all cases where personal injury compensation is paid. When a person receives an examination or treatment at an NHS hospital as a result of being involved in a road traffic or other accident and then makes a successful claim for personal injury compensation, the Secretary of State can require the insurance company to meet some of the treatment costs including any ambulance costs.

The Compensations Recovery Unit (CRU) undertakes the collection role on behalf of the Secretary of State. Once the insurance claim is settled and the CRU has recovered the NHS

---

[33] For more on research and development see:
www.dh.gov.uk/en/Policyandguidance/Researchanddevelopment/index.htm

charges, these will be paid to trusts. This amounted to £196m for the year ending 31 March 2011 including England, Wales, Scotland and ambulance trusts.

Provider to provider agreements

There may be localised arrangements between trusts to provide items such as facilities, services or staff to another healthcare provider – for example the cost of providing a staffed theatre session or several sessions of a consultant to another trust or provider. These arrangements are negotiated locally and should be covered by a contract.

National level clinical excellence awards

The Advisory Committee on Clinical Excellence Awards[34] (ACCEA) is an independent, advisory, non departmental body that is responsible for operating the national Clinical Excellence Awards Scheme. These clinical excellence awards are given to recognise and reward 'the exceptional contribution of NHS consultants' at a national level, 'over and above that normally expected in a job, to the values and goals of the NHS and to patient care'. The cost of these awards is funded centrally by the Department. Other 'Employer Based Awards' are awarded and funded by individual trusts.

Other commercial ventures

Many FTs are developing other commercial sources of income – for example, a repackaging unit for clinical instruments. When considering ventures of this type it should be borne in mind that FTs may, in the future, be subject to corporation tax above a certain level of turnover and in certain circumstances – see chapter 13.

Interest and investment income

Unlike other NHS trusts, FTs are allowed to retain surplus cash balances and invest these. Each FT is required to have a board approved policy for these investments which sets out: investment priorities; approved organisations it can invest in; limits per institution; maximum investment period, borrowing facilities and delegated powers. Given that FTs are now encouraged to retain and create surpluses knowledge of investment opportunities and treasury management is an important part of an FT finance function (see chapter 12).

8.4 Charitable Funds

Like other NHS trusts, FTs have charitable funds that can be used only for the purposes for which they were set up.

There are three main types of charitable funds recognised in law. These are:

- unrestricted funds – which may be spent at the discretion of the trustees in line with the charity's objectives

---

[34] Advisory Committee on Clinical Excellence Awards: www.advisorybodies.doh.gov.uk/accea/index.htm

- restricted income funds – which can only be spent in accordance with restrictions imposed by the donor when the funds were granted to, or raised for, the charity
- endowment funds – where capital funds are made available to a charity and trustees are legally required to invest or retain them. Endowment funds can be 'permanent' (trustees cannot spend the capital, only the income generated through its investment) or 'expendable' (capital can be converted to income).

Funds may also be 'designated' which means that trustees can earmark funds for a specific purpose. Designating funds can be useful where it is planned to build up balances through periodic transfers from unrestricted funds over time for a significant project or where funds are needed to meet ongoing costs (for example, staffing) to which formal commitments have been made.

There are five main sources of new money for charitable funds. These are:

- donations
- fundraising
- legacies
- investment income and interest
- grants.

Donations

Donations can be solicited (for example, through posters, leaflets or other appeals) or unsolicited (for example, where, at the end of a hospital stay, a patient asks how they can donate to the ward or hospital charity).

Donations of both types can be unrestricted or restricted. An unrestricted donation arises when for example, a patient or relative gives money 'for the hospital charity' or 'for the ward funds' without specifying how it should be used. A donation made in response to a fundraising leaflet, soliciting contributions for a general fund would also be unrestricted.

Fundraising

Fundraising income results from events (anything from coffee mornings and sponsored swims through to high profile celebrity events) and targeted appeals. If the money is sought for an explicit purpose (for example, if tickets or a poster for a charity dinner state 'all proceeds from this event will be used to buy monitors for the special care baby unit') then it must be used for that purpose and nothing else.

Legacies

Legacies (an amount of money left to the FT in a will) can be restricted or unrestricted depending on the terms on which the bequest is made.

Investment income and interest

Investment income and interest must be assigned to the fund that generates it.

Grants

Grants are usually restricted income given for a specific purpose. As well as the general principles which apply to the use of, and accounting for, restricted funds grants often have additional requirements attached.

For more about charitable funds refer to the HFMA's guide: NHS Charitable Funds: a Practical Guide or visit the Charity Commission's web site: www.charity-commission.gov.uk.

Chapter 9: Capital Funding

9.1 Introduction

One of the main differences between FTs and other trusts is the way in which they access capital funding.[35] This chapter focuses on the approach that FTs follow and the sources of funding available to them.

9.2 The Prudential Borrowing Code

In the interests of their long-term financial health, FTs strive to at least break even on the statement of comprehensive income. Indeed they may post surpluses for reinvestment in the future or alternatively post a planned deficit as part of a longer term balanced position. While not a statutory duty, 'managing the bottom-line' will always be a key corporate objective. However, measures of financial performance apply to FTs in line with their financial freedoms.

A key factor in an FT's long term financial planning is the effect of surpluses and deficits on its financial risk rating (FRR) – see section 5.3. The individual financial metrics that make up the FRR are set to require a modest level of surplus if a risk rating of 1 or 2 is to be avoided. The rationale for this approach is that surpluses are required to manage operational risks and ensure sufficient levels of finance for capital investment are made available in order to support the future development and improvement of services.

One of the most significant challenges facing FTs is the management of cash (for revenue or capital expenditure) and any associated borrowing. Monitor has published a prudential borrowing code that FTs must adhere to when applying for new borrowing.[36] This limits the *total* amount of money which an FT can borrow and aims to ensure that services provided to the public are not compromised by a foundation trust having more debt than it can manage.

The code itself takes account of generally accepted principles followed by financial institutions and focuses heavily on liquidity, meaning the strength of cash flow available to meet both dividend payments on opening and new Public Dividend Capital (PDC – see section 9.4), service interest and principal repayments on new loans. The measures are largely based around 'free cash flow' (FCF) or more specifically, 'revenue available for debt service' (RAfDS), which is defined as the operating surplus before depreciation and interest but excluding any exceptional transactions.

Without ensuring adequate levels of free cash flow FTs could find themselves in financial difficulties. For example, the situation might arise where new borrowing is entered into for a service development or expansion, which then fails to attract the expected level of patient

---

[35] The Department introduced a new capital regime for non FTs from 1 April 2007 which is similar to the approach followed by FTs.

[36] Prudential Borrowing Code for NHS Foundation Trusts, Monitor, 2009:
www.monitor-nhsft.gov.uk/sites/default/files/Prudential%20Borrowing%20Code%20April%202009_0.pdf

income because demand falls, either through a lack of partnership working or due to a failure to properly assess the risk. FTs must therefore ensure that their financial performance is monitored closely. Monitor has powers to intervene if an FT fails financially (see section 5.4).

An FT must remain within the prudential borrowing limit (PBL) set by Monitor based on its ability to repay any loans it enters into. The PBL is the *maximum* amount of debt the FT can have outstanding at any point in time and is specified in the terms of its authorisation. It is reviewed at least annually in conjunction with the annual plan and can be varied upwards or downwards. There are two parts to the PBL neither of which may be breached:

- the maximum amount of cumulative long term borrowing that is, long term loans which will include any outstanding debt relating to a PFI or Local Improvement Finance Trust (LIFT) contract
- the working capital facility that is, short term borrowing (see section 12.6).

Long term borrowing is governed by a two-tier system

- tier 1 limit is based on the annual plan submission
- tier 2 limit which may be available to accommodate affordable major investments including PFI schemes.

The Prudential Borrowing Code for NHS foundation trusts states that 'When an NHSFT is planning a transaction that would exceed its Tier 1 limit it is required to submit a request to Monitor for a Tier 2 limit, which, if approved, will replace the Tier 1 limit. Monitor will consider each application for a Tier 2 limit on a case-by-case basis'.[37]

Financial ratios are used to calculate the FT's performance against its PBL and help ensure that all borrowing remains affordable. The tier 1 ratios are:

- **minimum dividend cover** ($>1\times$) – this ratio effectively requires that an FT has sufficient FCF to meet its annual dividend payment to the Department (at least once) calculated as 3.5% of the average value of its net assets. The formula is: RAfDS less interest divided by annual dividend payable
- **minimum interest cover** ($>3\times$) – this financial constraint is the interest coverage ratio measured by the number of times that RAfDS covers interest repayments in any one year. The formula is: RAfDS divided by maximum annual interest
- **minimum debt service cover** ($>2\times$) – this ratio requires that RAfDS is sufficient to meet all interest and principal payments on long term borrowing, measured as RAfDS divided by maximum annual debt service
- **maximum debt service to revenue** ($<2.5\%$) – this ratio seeks to ensure that the cost of servicing debt and loans is no more than 2.5% of a trust's total revenue. It is measured by calculating maximum annual debt service divided by revenue.

---

[37] Prudential Borrowing Code for NHS Foundation Trusts, Monitor, 2009: www.regulator-nhsft.gov.uk/publications.php

The tier 2 ratios are reviewed annually based on the projections made in the FT's annual plan. The tier 2 limit is subject to a maximum cap determined through the same ratio tests as for tier 1 but with revised thresholds. The thresholds for both tier 1 and tier 2 ratios are shown in the table below:

Ratio	Tier 1 Threshold	Tier 2 Threshold
Minimum dividend cover	>1×	1×
Minimum interest cover	>3×	>2×
Minimum debt service cover	>2×	>1.5×
Maximum debt service to revenue	<2.5%	<10%

9.3 Affordability/Planning

The PBL is initially determined from the 'service development strategy' submitted as part of the FT application, and is reviewed at least annually as part of the annual plan submission.

'Borrowing' includes loans from the FT financing facility (see section 9.5), commercial borrowing and finance leases, PFI and LIFT schemes but excludes PDC which is classed as equity in this instance.

The PBL is calculated using the plan figures and is set so as to ensure that the financial ratios continue to be met. It is important to understand that the FRR is a key factor in determining the PBL, since any significant reduction in this figure in year could lead to a reduction in PBL in year (see section 5.3 for more on the FRR).

A worked example is shown below:

The table below shows the income and expenditure plan for an FT with a risk rating of 5. Net assets are valued at £114.3m and when multiplied by the Department's required rate of return of 3.5% results in a dividend payment due of £4m.

Income/expenditure – original plan	£000
Income	200,000
Pay and non-pay costs	(189,000)
Depreciation	(7,000)
Operating surplus	4,000
Finance costs:	
PDC repaid to the Department	(4,000)
Surplus/(deficit)	0

The planned statement of cash flows (see below) prior to considering any new venture, shows a capital spend of £10m.

To finance the capital programme, the FT will receive £3m in additional public dividend capital (PDC) from the Department and its overall cash position will be unchanged.

Statement of cash flows	£000
Operating surplus	4,000
Add back: non-cash expense	
Depreciation	7,000
Net cash generated from operations	11,000
Cash flows from investing activities:	
Capital spend	(10,000)
Net cash flows from investing activities	(10,000)
Cash flows from financing activities	
PDC repaid	(4,000)
Additional PDC from Department	3,000
Net cash flows from financing activities	(1,000)
Increase/(decrease) in cash	0

The first test of this plan is to ensure that no financial ratios have been breached. The relevant figures are:

Revenue available for debt service	£000
Operating surplus	4,000
Add back: non-cash expense	
Depreciation	7,000
Revenue available for debt service	11,000
PDC repaid	(4,000)
Total Assets [note: not net assets]	120,000

Using these figures, the ratios for the above plan are:

Prudential Borrowing Code	
Minimum Dividend Cover (>1×)	2.75
Minimum Interest Cover (>3×)	n/a
Minimum Debt Service Cover (>2×)	n/a
Maximum Debt Service to Revenue (<2.5%)	n/a

The only ratio of relevance here is the minimum dividend cover – the other ratios require the FT to have a loan before they can be meaningfully calculated.

Within its application and five year planning statement, the FT requested and was granted a prudential borrowing limit of £48m. It does not, however, need to use this level of borrowing, but rather has satisfied Monitor that this level of debt could be taken on without breaching the ratios.

An opportunity has arisen to spend additional capital on expanding capacity for day case/inpatient activity and under PbR this will attract an average reimbursement of £2,000 per case. Projected activity is 2,000 cases per year with gross income of £4m (£2,000 × 2,000). Pay and non-pay costs are anticipated to be £3.26m.

The FT is choosing to exercise its prudential borrowing limit and applies to the FT financing facility for a loan based on the parameters shown below:

Loan profile	£000
Loan value	5,000
Interest rate	4.8%
Term of repayment	10 years
Useful life	10 years
Value at end of life	0
Repayment profile	Equal instalments of principal (EIP)
Total loan repayments, per annum	740
Interest in year 1	240
Principal repaid in year 1	500
Depreciation costs per year	500

The FT must satisfy a number of stakeholders that this venture is affordable and one that will deliver substantial benefits in terms of reduced waiting times, improved access and enhanced quality. From a financial view, the first step is to amend the opening plan to determine the combined impact on income and expenditure.

Income/expenditure	Original Plan £000	New Venture £000	Amended Plan £000
Income	200,000	4,000	204,000
Pay and non-pay costs	(189,000)	(3,260)	(192,260)
Depreciation	(7,000)	(500)	(7,500)
Operating surplus	4,000	240	4,240
PDC repaid	(4,000)	–	(4,000)
Interest on new loan	–	(240)	(240)
Net surplus/(deficit)	0	0	0

As well as a revised income and expenditure plan, the statement of cash flows is updated to show the incremental changes. Capital expenditure is increased by 50% (£10m + £5m) and the cash outflows associated with servicing the new loan are included.

There is no increase in cash since the loan term is the same as the useful life of the investment – so principal repayments equal depreciation.

Statement of cash flows	Original Plan £000	New Venture £000	Amended Plan £000
Operating surplus	4,000	240	4,240
Add back: non-cash expense Depreciation	7,000	500	7,500
Net cash flows from operations	11,000	740	11,740
Cash flows from investing activities: Capital spend	(10,000)	(5,000)	(15,000)
Net cash flows from investing activities	(10,000)	(5,000)	(15,000)
Cash flows from financing activities: PDC repaid	(4,000)	–	(4,000)
Interest on new loan	–	(240)	(240)
Additional PDC from Department	3,000	–	3,000
New loan	–	5,000	5,000
Loan principal repaid	–	(500)	(500)
Net cash flows from financing activities	(1,000)	4,260	3,260
Increase/(decrease) in cash	0	0	0

A major factor in the decision making process concerns the impact on the trust's ratios.

The relevant figures are:

Revenue available for debt service	Original Plan £000	New Venture £000	Amended Plan £000
Operating surplus	4,000	240	4,240
Add back: non-cash expense Depreciation	7,000	500	7,500
Revenue available for debt service	11,000	740	11,740
Income	200,000	4,000	204,000
PDC repaid	(4,000)	–	(4,000)
Interest on new loan	–	(240)	(240)
Loan principal repaid	–	(500)	(500)
Total Assets	120,000	4,500	124,500

The ratios for the above new venture and the amended plan are:

Prudential Borrowing Code	Original Plan £000	New Venture £000	Amended Plan £000
Minimum Dividend Cover (>1×)	2.75	n/a	2.94
Minimum Interest Cover (>2×)	n/a	3.08	49
Minimum Debt Service Cover (>1.5×)	n/a	1.00	15.86
Maximum Debt Service to Revenue (<10%)	n/a	18.5%	0.36%

From the above we can see that the new venture on its own breaches two of the four ratio tests:

- minimum debt service cover is below the required level of 1.5
- the total amount of debt exceeds 10% of the total income.

However, this new venture will be considered based on the impact on the organisation's entire financial position. On this basis, there is sufficient flexibility in the FT's finances to meet all ratio requirements. Moreover, the proposal provides a break-even position.

In practice, there would be a number of other financial tests associated with the decision. They include 'sensitivity analysis' to determine the risk associated with the new venture – for example, if income fell by 10%–15% but costs only reduced by 8%, the FT may breach its ratios. Also, a series of option appraisals (including discounted cash flows over a number of years) need to be evaluated to determine the most effective use of capital.

9.4 Public Dividend Capital Funding

Whereas the primary source of funding for an FT is likely to be borrowing, it is still possible that schemes in existence at authorisation, and some central initiatives could be funded via PDC from the Department.

If an FT has agreed PDC funding with the Department, then a 'PDC Limit' is set by the Department. This is similar to a 'cash based capital resource limit (CRL)',[38] in that an FT may only access the PDC once it has fully utilised its own internal cash generated through retained depreciation and sale proceeds from the disposal of non-current assets.

For example, an FT may have agreed £4m PDC funding for a particular capital project but if its retained depreciation is £3m and its operational capital plans are only £2m, then the PDC Limit will be calculated as follows:

---

[38] A CRL is an expenditure limit determined by the Department for each non FT NHS organisation limiting the amount that may be expended on capital purchases.

	£m
Operational capital plan	2
Capital project	4
Total	**6**
Retained Depreciation	(3)
PDC Limit	3

The remaining £1m of PDC originally agreed is 'lost'. To avoid losing PDC funding in this way FTs need to consider utilising their retained depreciation cash. However, this may not fit with the organisation's wider financial strategy. In particular, FTs may wish to adopt an aggressive working capital strategy to improve liquidity through retained depreciation cash, or indeed may wish to manage the cash implications of a financial recovery plan through slippage in capital investment.

9.5 Sources of Borrowing

The main source of operational capital funding is from internally generated resources – that is, retained depreciation, asset sales and cash surpluses. Larger schemes will require an FT to borrow within its PBL ratios as outlined above.

Although some FTs have already sought funding from the commercial sector, it was envisaged initially that the market would be too immature to attract significant interest from commercial lenders and that – in the absence of an agreed insolvency regime and asset security – it may prove expensive. For this reason the Department formed the FT Financing Facility (FTFF) – this operates at 'arms length' from the Department and makes loan decisions based on the ability of the FT 'to pay back the money, not on the basis of a policy judgement'.[39] Loans are made available at a preferential rate (equivalent to the national loans fund rate) for core business (that is, to 'to fund development to essential protected services'), and at a market rate for commercial developments or 'non-protected activity'.

9.6 Public Private Partnerships – the Private Finance Initiative

Introduction

Another source of funding for capital projects involves working in partnership with the private sector – most commonly using the Private Finance Initiative or PFI.

What is the Private Finance Initiative?

Private Finance Initiative (PFI) is a government scheme set up as part of the strategy to deliver high quality public services by having the right infrastructure in place. The PFI is a mechanism for funding major capital investments without immediate recourse to public money and allows

---

[39] NHS Foundation Trusts Information Guide – Financial Freedoms, Department of Health, 2004: available via the Department's web site (use the search function – key in 'financial freedoms'): www.dh.gov.uk

public services such as the NHS to raise funds for capital projects from commercial organisations. Private companies are contracted to design and build the assets needed which are then 'leased back' to the public sector, usually over a period of around 30 years. Many NHS trusts have entered into PFI agreements in order to fund major capital projects which they would have otherwise been unable to afford such as the building of new wings, buildings or even entire hospitals.

Under the PFI responsibility for the design, construction, maintenance, operation and financing of capital assets rests with the private sector. The public sector focus is on defining the standards of service required – the private sector partner then decides how it can best deliver a service to meet those standards. The public sector client pays for the service when it becomes operational and the payment is linked to satisfactory service provision. Payment takes the form of a unitary charge paid to the PFI provider. Financing the asset construction is the responsibility of the PFI provider and often utilises a range of funding mechanisms, including loans, equity or bonds.

Since the introduction of International Financial Reporting Standards (IFRS) to the NHS in 2009, the way in which a PFI service is accounted for has changed. Previously an asset provided under a PFI service contract was not deemed to be owned by the public sector organisation and did not therefore appear on its balance sheet. This reduced the need for public sector capital and the public sector borrowing requirement.

With the application of IFRS, PFI and Local Improvement Finance Trusts (LIFT) schemes are brought onto the public sector organisation's balance sheet or statement of financial position as it is now known. As a finance lease, the scheme must be accounted for as an asset with depreciation charges as if the asset were owned by the trust and a liability recorded for the amount of the lease outstanding. Therefore as with any other non-current asset, depreciation charges are incurred. In addition, although the cash leaving the organisation to the private partner is unchanged, the unitary payment is now split into its component parts, each of which is accounted for separately.

PFI in the NHS

PFI schemes involve creating partnerships between the public and private sectors that allow the NHS to focus on the provision of high quality clinical care to patients while the private sector provides investment to help deliver the modernisation agenda.

In essence, a PFI project is a contract between an NHS body and a private sector organisation for the provision of services over an agreed contract period. The private sector organisation will normally be in the form of a special purpose vehicle (SPV) or special purpose company (SPC) established specifically for the project. The SPV may consist of a construction company, a facilities management company and a financing organisation. The exact composition varies for each project. Similarly the length of the contract depends on the nature of the service to be provided – a new hospital for example may have a contract period of 30 years.

The contract will set out in detail the obligations of each party. The development of a PFI project must follow a prescribed process in the NHS and comply with EU procurement guidance.

PFI and FTs

The Department and Monitor have issued guidance as to their relative roles in the assessment of the affordability of PFI projects.[40] This guidance is reproduced below.

Monitor will consider the potential implication from a risk perspective and where it considers that the proposal may give rise to too much risk it will be unlikely to recommend to the Department or the Treasury that the proposal be allowed to proceed.

Ultimately, it is the role of the FT board of directors to approve or reject the proposal. More detail on their role, and that of other parties, is set out below.

Roles and Responsibilities in the Approval of NHS Foundation Trust PFI Schemes

Strategic health authorities/primary care trusts	The key role currently played by the SHA and PCTs will be to confirm that they want the services proposed by the NHS foundation trust in the planned geographical location and that the activity levels proposed in the PFI business case are realistic. Without such confirmation, the income assumptions cannot be supported and the project would not be viable.
NHS foundation trust board of directors	The role of the NHS foundation trust (NHSFT) board of directors is ultimately to approve or reject the proposal. We would expect an NHSFT board to treat a PFI scheme in the same way as any other major investment. Monitor has issued detailed best practice advice on appraising major investments in its publication Risk Evaluation for Investment Decisions by NHS Foundation Trusts.
	Further, Monitor's Compliance Framework gives details as to how they will deal with major investments including PFI schemes. NHSFT boards will be expected to comply with immediate effect.
Monitor	Monitor's role is to review proposals for major investments and to ensure that the financial viability of the NHSFT will not be undermined if the transaction proceeds. In carrying out such a review Monitor will not approve or reject the scheme. That is the role of the board of the NHSFT. Monitor does expect the board, however, to take into consideration the findings of the Monitor review and the likely impact on the published financial risk rating (FRR) if the scheme were to go ahead.
	Monitor's role will be to calculate an FRR for the first two years in which the full unitary payment is payable by the NHSFT. The FRR will be calculated under both the base case scenario and a reasonable downside case. Where the FRR for either case is 1 or 2

---

[40] Roles and Responsibilities in the Approval of NHS Foundation Trust PFI Schemes, Monitor and the DH, June 2007: www.monitor-nhsft.gov.uk/home/our-publications/browse-category/guidance-foundation-trusts

	in either of those years, Monitor would not expect the NHSFT board to approve the scheme. In any event, taken together with the fact that Department of Health will not provide a Deed of Safeguard (see below) for schemes with a FRR of 1 or 2, it means schemes so rated will not be able to progress. In calculating the FRR, Monitor will review the key revenue and cost assumptions used in the financial projections. These key assumptions will be stress tested through sensitivity analysis in calculating the FRR. In concluding on financial assumptions Monitor would expect to discuss activity assumptions with the NHSFT and proposed key commissioners of the services being provided through the scheme. All other key assumptions would be the subject of discussion between Monitor, the NHSFT and the Department.
Department of Health and HM Treasury (HMT)	The Department's guidance on delegated limits is not applicable to NHSFTs. However, the Department and HMT have a key role to play where a Deed of Safeguard is required. This is currently the case for the majority of PFI transactions since without the Deed of Safeguard there would be no commercial deal. As above, where the FRR is either 1 or 2 the Department or HMT will not issue a Deed of Safeguard. For the purpose of the issue of the Deed of Safeguard, the Department and HMT have set out their requirements. This includes adherence to the standard PFI contract; specified funding structures; payment mechanisms; the requisite level of due diligence before approval can be granted and a duly approved full business case (FBC). The precise requirements are available from the Department's Private Finance Unit.
Sequence	The sequence of reviews is as follows: 1. Agree service proposals and activity levels with service commissioners 2. Monitor's review and FRR. 3. Deed of Safeguard review by Department/HMT

Chapter 10: Payment by Results

10.1 What is Payment by Results?

Payment by Results (PbR) is the system for reimbursing healthcare providers in England for the costs of providing treatment. PbR is based around the use of a prospective, tariff-based system that links a preset price to a defined measure of output or activity. It replaced the traditional approach where commissioners and providers negotiated annual patient service agreements focussing heavily on the unit cost of treatment. Instead there is a single national price list or 'tariff' for services applicable to all providers of NHS care. The tariff is based on the current costs of all providers analysed by healthcare resource groups (HRGs). HRGs group conditions that are clinically similar and require similar resources for treatment and care. They are often referred to as the 'currency' that is used for commissioning. They have been developed by clinicians in order to provide clinically meaningful groups of conditions and treatments which require similar levels of resource.

Not all healthcare activities are covered by PbR however, significant steps are being taken to expand its scope. Some areas of acute care remain outside of PbR at present, for example critical care and chemotherapy services. A typical large acute trust may have 20% of its prices determined at a local level (non-mandatory tariffs) through negotiation with commissioners for services outside the scope of PbR.

PbR involves payment for services at the full national tariff rate and a reduction in payments for underperformance also at the full national rate. Therefore, significant incentives have been created to ensure delivery of baseline activity and to maximise the use of spare and additional capacity.

A market forces factor is applied to allow for the fact that the cost base varies across the country – this adjustment is paid direct to providers (see section 8.2).

10.2 The Impact on FTs

Acute FTs were able to adopt PbR a year before other NHS trusts. This early introduction along with legally binding contracts between commissioners and FTs has changed the approach taken to service planning and delivery. For example with a national tariff, annual service agreement planning should focus on quality and effective delivery of health services rather than protracted negotiations on unit prices. PbR arrangements however continue to allow for some local flexibility to encourage innovation. As significant areas of acute care are still outside of PbR, it is still necessary for local price discussions to take place, but not to the same extent as before.

10.3 The Code of Conduct

In recognition of the fact that PbR can be effective only if there are constructive relationships between all the parties involved, the Department developed a Code of Conduct which aims to:

- 'establish core principles, with some ground rules for organisational behaviour, and expectations as to how the system should operate
- minimise disputes, as well as guide the resolution of them'.

All NHS bodies operating PbR must comply with the Code, and boards of all other organisations are encouraged to adopt it.

As far as FTs are concerned, William Moyes, the former Executive Chairman of Monitor has said:

'We have seen with the first NHS foundation trusts how PbR provides powerful incentives for efficiency; but it is essential that the relationship between commissioner and provider is clearly defined and that both parties live up to their responsibilities. The Code will help ensure that happens and so we welcome it.'

The Code focuses on the behaviour and responsibilities of all those involved in PbR including commissioners, providers and other organisations. It also looks at:

- how information should be shared
- billing and payment
- activity specification, demand management and capacity
- referrals and treatment thresholds
- innovation to improve access to, or quality of, services
- enforcement.

10.4 The Future of PbR

The coalition government and the Department have clearly identified the future direction of PbR and the national tariff. There have been a number of key developments in the last two years as it is used to incentivise behaviours and actions, to support healthcare policy and the strategic aims of the NHS. As policy and objectives develop and change over time, so must PbR. These key developments are outlined below:

Quality

Following the publication of Lord Darzi's review *High Quality Care for All* there was a renewed focus on quality of services to patients. This resulted in the initial introduction of four best practice tariffs in 2010/11.

Best practice tariffs aim to bring together quality and efficiency by rewarding high quality care. Rather than being set at the national average cost of delivering the procedures concerned, they reflect the costs of delivering best practice, for example by undertaking cholecystectomies as a day case procedure or admitting stroke patients directly to a dedicated stroke unit. The standard tariff (that is, *not* best practice) is set lower than the best practice tariff price to encourage providers to adopt best practice patient pathways. Those providers failing to deliver best practice will attract a lower payment for their activity. As this is applied across the NHS in England, national improvements in the quality of care in these areas should materialise.

The range of best practice tariffs has been expanded in 2011/12 and 2012/13 and this likely to continue in the coming years.

In addition healthcare providers are rewarded for specific improvements to services under the Commissioning for Quality and Innovation (CQUIN) policy whereby a percentage of contract income is attached to local quality improvement goals for example, through improving the effectiveness of discharge information (see section 8.2).

Scope

Although community, mental health and ambulance services are currently outside the scope of PbR, significant steps are being taken to introduce a tariff for community and mental health services. A new currency for adult mental health services was made available for local use in 2010/11. The government is mandating these currencies – based on care clusters – from 2012/13, although prices will still be set locally. Developed following clinical guidance and successful pilots across England, care clusters reflect a patient's needs over a given period of time.

Currencies continue to be introduced for a number of other services to increase the coverage of PbR, although prices will be for local negotiation between commissioners and providers. The introduction of a national currency provides a common basis for agreeing contracts alongside local flexibility to fit with the financial situation of local health economies.

Influence

Increasingly, the tariff is being used to influence the behaviour of those commissioning and providing services to patients and to support the overall strategic aims of the NHS. There are two clear examples of this in the way PbR has been developed to reduce emergency admissions to hospitals.

Emergency activity

The way in which emergency inpatient activity was paid for by commissioners was changed in 2010/11. Providers of emergency services are paid at full tariff for the number of patients admitted to hospital as an emergency up to the value of the activity recorded for the financial year 2008/09 priced at the tariff for the current year.

However, admissions over and above this baseline are only paid at a marginal or per patient rate of 30% of tariff. Therefore, health economies where the emergency admissions consistently exceed the baseline should aim to redesign services and manage patient demand for those services. In practice, the financial incentive clearly sits with the acute trusts, so they will need to find ways to engage with local PCTs to help solve the problem. The additional money that the PCT would have spent on paying for the activity at full tariff (that is, 70%) is handed over to the strategic health authority to fund changes in the way emergency services are provided.

Readmissions to hospital

An early change announced soon after the coalition government came to power was that service providers would no longer receive any further payment for a patient admitted within

30 days of their discharge following a planned or non-elective admission. In other words, hospitals will be penalised if the patient is readmitted within a 30 day period if the readmission is related to the original reason for care.

This came into effect from 1 April 2011 and aims to reduce the number of emergency admissions to hospital by up to 25% – so if the readmission rate was 10% last year, the threshold will be set at 7.5%. A number of patient groups are excluded from the rule for example, maternity, cancer and paediatric patients.

Pathway tariffs

The Department has already committed to the future introduction of a tariff to reflect patient pathways. This is to apply initially to maternity services where the pathway combines care in both community and secondary settings, with some elements of the pathway paid for under the old style block contracts while hospital interventions are covered by PbR. A pathway tariff will also be introduced in 2012/13 for paediatric diabetes.

Introducing a tariff to cover the whole of the patient pathway should facilitate the delivery of the right care to patients in the right setting but as cost effectively as possible.

Future roles and responsibilities

As far as the mechanics of PbR are concerned the government is proposing that in future prices will be set by Monitor in its role as economic regulator. The intention is that it will work with the NHS Commissioning Board to decide which services should be subject to national tariffs. The development of currencies for pricing and payment will also be a joint responsibility, although the Commissioning Board will have primary responsibility for determining currencies.

Chapter 11: Financial Planning, Accounting and Reporting

11.1 The Annual Plan

Monitor's Compliance Framework requires each FT to submit a forward looking plan (annual plan) to the regulator by 31 May each year. Monitor also updates its Compliance Framework with the requirements of the annual plan to incorporate amendments and additions resulting from consultation exercises, particularly in relation to clinical quality, service line reporting and the financial risk ratings.

In practice this means that each year FTs must prepare and submit a three year plan (current year and two future years). This plan should contain, as a minimum, the following information as specified in the Compliance Framework:

- strategic priorities
- forecast financial and service performance
- details of any major risks to compliance with its authorisation and how these will be addressed.

For full details see chapter 2 of the latest Compliance Framework.[41]

Monitor's Code of Governance also makes clear that the board of directors should present a balanced and understandable assessment of the NHS foundation trust's financial position and prospects. The board of directors should present its annual accounts and reports as well as quality accounts at the annual general meeting to allow members and governors to evaluate its performance. The members and governors must also be 'presented with, for consideration, the annual plan, both qualitative and quantitative at the general meeting. The governors can expect to be consulted on the development of forward plans for the trust and any significant changes to the delivery of the trust's business plan'.

Monitor publishes guidance to help FTs develop their annual plans which is updated annually.

A typical annual plan prepared by an FT will consist of the following:

- executive summary
- introduction
- overall plan commentary including:
  - strategy over the plan period and delivery milestones
  - summary of national and local factors
  - summary financial commentary
  - financial plans covering
    - income

- ○ service developments
- ○ activity
- ○ costs
- ○ workforce
- ○ capital programmes
- ○ clinical plans including quality accounts
- ○ regulatory requirements
- ○ leadership arrangements and succession plans where appropriate
- membership report
  - ○ membership size and movement
  - ○ membership analysis
  - ○ turnout at elections
  - ○ membership plans for the future
- board statement covering
  - ○ risk
  - ○ service performance
  - ○ clinical quality
  - ○ compliance with the terms of authorisation
  - ○ board roles, structures and capacity
- financial projections for the current year and three future years
  - ○ income statement
  - ○ balance sheet/statement of financial position
  - ○ cash flow statement
- annual update to mandatory services and mandatory education and training.

It is important that the production of the annual plan is not regarded as solely the responsibility of the finance function. Although it contains a good deal of financial information and projections, further information must be collated within the organisation – for example, service and business development, human resources, information and estates to ensure that financial forecasts closely mirror the organisation's service planning assumptions.

The annual plan also requires information from outside the FT. In particular, any changes to the tariff and commissioning intentions from major commissioners are needed. This can be difficult to obtain as their approach to planning may be less detailed than is required for populating the FT's plans.

From a practical perspective, it is essential that the FT uses its own activity model as a starting point for the annual plan. This can then be adjusted for known changes including future commissioning intentions. Outputs from the activity model can be 'dropped' into a financial model which generates a financial plan in the format of both the FT's management and financial accounts.

As well as setting out a strategic plan, FTs must consider the detailed implications of their plan for example, a plan to develop a particular service will have implications for the level of capital spend, tariff income levels etc. and these would be incorporated into each year's projections. In addition, there will be technical and legislative changes to be reflected.

This annual financial projection, once finalised, can be fed into the FT's finance system and then used to generate the monthly monitoring data in both the financial management and accounting formats to enable regular monitoring and reporting.

11.2 The Annual Accounts

Statutory requirement

All NHS bodies have a statutory duty to produce annual accounts as set out in the NHS Act 2006. The form and content of the annual accounts is prescribed by Monitor (with the approval of the Treasury). As with all NHS organisations, FTs must follow International Financial Reporting Standards (IFRS). The production of the statutory annual accounts is the principal means by which FTs discharge their accountability to taxpayers and users of services for their stewardship of public money.

NHS accounting framework

NHS bodies are expected to adhere to the accounting standards issued or adopted by the Accounting Standards Board (ASB).[42] However, the government has the final say on how these standards are applied to the public sector, including NHS bodies. The Treasury has developed a Financial Reporting Manual setting out how accounting standards should be implemented in the public sector. For FTs, Monitor produces an NHS Foundation Trust Annual Reporting Manual (ARM) which is broadly consistent with the Treasury's manual with any divergences being first approved by the Treasury.

Monitor's ARM provides a summary of extant accounting standards and their applicability to FTs. FTs may need to refer to the standards themselves if a more detailed understanding is required. Accounting standards are intended to provide a framework for best practice and the common disclosure of information. They provide the benchmark against which an organisation's audited accounts are compared and judged.

Accounts format and timetable

The Annual Reporting Manual (which is updated on an annual basis) specifies the format and timing of FTs' annual accounts and schedules, which consist of:

- a set of consolidation schedules (FTCs)
- a set of annual accounts.

The format of the FTCs is determined by Monitor but FTs have the freedom to adapt the format of their accounts provided it remains consistent with the FTCs. As well as preparing the statutory annual accounts, FTs must complete consolidation schedules which are used by Monitor to produce a summary of all FT accounts. The use of consolidation schedules also facilitates the preparation of whole of government accounts (WGA). The accounts and FTCs are submitted to Monitor and the external auditors simultaneously.

---

[42] The Accounting Standards Board web site can be found at www.frc.org.uk/asb

An FTs' annual accounts consist of:

- the foreword to the accounts
- the four primary statements:
  - the statement of comprehensive income
  - the statement of financial position
  - the statement of changes in taxpayers' equity
  - the statement of cash flows
- the notes to the accounts
- statements and certificates:
  - the accounting officer's statement of responsibilities
  - the annual governance statement
  - the remuneration report
  - the auditor's opinion and certificate.

Once the annual accounts have been prepared they must be audited. Once audited and the necessary amendments made, the board of directors is required to formally adopt the accounts. The certificates are signed by the chief executive at the same time. The auditor then signs the audit report.

The ARM sets out the timetable for completing the accounts and audit.

Quality accounts

Lord Darzi's report *High Quality Care for All* (June 2008) proposed that all providers of NHS healthcare services should produce a 'quality account' that is, an annual report to the public about the quality of services delivered. The Health Act 2009 has made this a statutory requirement. Foundation trusts have been at the forefront of the development of quality accounts. Quality accounts were introduced in 2008/09 for the first time and 2009/10 annual plans were the first to include them. Foundation trusts were required to identify their priorities for improvement and what indicators they would be using to measure their performance against these priorities.

The introduction of quality accounts aims to encourage boards to assess quality across all services provided by the organisation whilst seeking continuous quality improvement over the longer term. Through transparent reporting, they should provide assurance to the public, commissioners and members that the board of directors is regularly scrutinising each service provided.

Quality accounts are made available to the public and comprise a number of mandatory elements as follows:

- a statement on quality from the chief executive (or equivalent) of the organisation
- priorities for improvement and statements of assurance from the board – as well as comparing actual performance to the previous year's priorities, the forward looking section shows clearly the plans for quality improvement, the reasons for choosing these priorities, while demonstrating how the FT is developing capacity and capability to deliver the quality improvements

- a section providing an overview of the quality of care provided by the FT during the previous year against pre-determined indicators which must include:
  - at least 3 indicators for patient safety
  - at least 3 indicators for clinical effectiveness
  - at least 3 indicators for patient experience
  - performance against national priorities.

The directors must also include a signed statement in relation to the way in which the quality account has been prepared. The audit committee should seek assurance as to the way in which the quality account has been prepared.

Quality accounts require external independent assurance, similar to that applied to the annual report and accounts. This means that the quality accounts will be audited by the FT's external auditors and an audit opinion published.

11.3 The Annual Report

FTs are required to produce an annual report which must be published with either the full set of audited accounts or summary financial statements and include quality accounts and reports. The annual report is primarily a narrative document similar to the directors' report described in the Companies Act, but with additional information reflecting the FT's position in the community. The report gives an account of activities, performance and achievements over the last financial year.

Although the exact format and content of the annual report is left to the discretion of the FT, there are mandatory items which must be included and are specified in the FT Annual Reporting Manual.

The annual report and accounts must be approved by the board of directors prior to submission to Monitor. FTs are required to lay their report and accounts (the full accounts – not summary financial statements) before Parliament themselves. This has to be done before the summer recess.[43]

The annual report and accounts must also be presented to the board of governors. This meeting should be convened within a reasonable timescale after the end of the financial year, but must not be before the FT has laid its annual report and accounts before Parliament.

The content of the annual report

The format and content of the annual report is individual to each organisation. A typical annual report is likely to include the following:

- forewords by the chairman and chief executive
- membership details

---

[43] See Monitor's Annual Reporting Manual 2010/11 for full details: www.monitor-nhsft.gov.uk

- details of the board of directors and board of governors
- details of the audit committee and nominations committee
- performance of individual directorates and business units
- information in relation to sustainability and climate change
- operating financial review
- remuneration report
- annual governance statement
- independent auditor's report
- annual accounts/summary financial statements
- quality accounts/reports.

11.4 In Year Reporting and Monitoring – External

As we've seen, FTs must submit an annual plan to Monitor, including three years of financial forecasts, service development and membership strategies.

Initially, an FT must submit quarterly performance reports to Monitor setting out its financial information for the last quarter and year to date along with a commentary on any variances or changes. However, as the compliance regime is risk-based, well-governed high-performing FTs are given space to exercise their freedoms and may, in time, be required to report less frequently. Where FTs are experiencing significant financial or service problems, oversight is more intensive and monthly reporting may be required.

FTs must report to Monitor 'any material, actual or prospective changes which may affect their ability to comply with any aspect of their authorisation' – for example, any plans to vary mandatory service provision or an adverse auditors' report.

The main contents of the quarterly submissions are:

Finance

- the four primary financial statements – actual performance versus that planned for the current and previous quarter
- a financial commentary including explanations of variances and any reforecast as needed
- the anticipated maintenance of a financial risk rating of at least 3 or above in the next four quarters
- forward financial indicators to highlight the potential for any future material financial breaches of authorisation. This includes the use of the FT's working capital facility in the previous quarter and whether the FT has an interim finance director over more than one quarter end (see section 5.3).

Governance

- certifications by the board that targets have been met (such as those for Methicillin Resistant Staphylococcus Aureus (MRSA) and clostridium difficile)
- exception reports which may relate to any issue which may affect the FT's compliance with the terms of its authorisation for example, any requirement for working capital in breach of prudential borrowing limits

- board statement on quality
- results of any governor elections
- reports of any changes to the board of directors or board of governors.

More details about what Monitor expects from FTs is set out in chapter 5 of this guide and in the latest Compliance Framework.[44]

FTs must also submit annual reference costs to the Department. Reference costs are collected from all NHS providers and capture the total cost to each organisation of its patient contacts in the previous financial year. The data is used to inform the national tariff under Payment by Results. To ensure consistency across all providers, the Department specifies the definitions and approach that must be used – see the Department's website for more details.[45]

11.5 In Year Reporting and Monitoring – Internal

Reporting to budget holders

The reporting of performance against the financial plan and the corrective action taken as a result is an essential element of financial management in the NHS. Reporting to budget holders should be in sufficient detail to ensure that all significant variances are identified so that any necessary corrective action can be taken.

While the nature and format of budget monitoring information will vary between different levels in the organisation, the over-riding requirement is that the information is timely and accurate. To ensure accurate monthly financial reports, financial commitments should be recognised as soon as possible and be reflected in the monthly reports. Without accurate budget reporting at budget holder level, costs cannot be effectively controlled.

Budget monitoring information is produced at a range of levels, allowing managers to see not only summary performance, but also the performance of individual departments and teams. The exact nature of this reporting depends on the organisation's management structure. These reports on revenue and expenditure are often referred to as the 'management accounts'.

FTs should also ensure that budget holders receive regular training so that they have sufficient skills to undertake the task of effective budget management.

It is important to note that the development of service line reporting and management has an impact on FTs' approaches to budget setting and monitoring (see section 5.3).

Reporting to boards

The board of directors needs financial information so that it can properly direct the organisation. This information has to be accurate and timely so that early and corrective action

---

[44] Compliance Framework, Monitor, 2011/12: www.monitor-nhsft.gov.uk
[45] Reference costs – information and guidance is available from:
www.dh.gov.uk/en/Managingyourorganisation/Financeandplanning/NHScostingmanual/index.htm

can be taken where necessary. The form, content and frequency of financial reports will vary between FTs and it is for each board of directors to decide what it needs to receive in this area. The types of information which may be reported to the board of directors include:

- performance against the achievement of statutory duties and healthcare and service targets including action plans for the resolution of any breaches
- performance against quality indicators
- performance against governance and financial risk ratings
- in-year revenue and expenditure position and year-end forecasts, including an analysis of financial risks, the likelihood of them arising and how they will be managed
- in-year performance against the indicators of forward financial risk
- activity levels linked to financial data
- progress on the achievement of any cost improvement programmes and financial recovery plans
- statement of financial position
- statement of cash flows and cash flow forecast
- working capital position
- losses
- performance of outsourced services
- progress against internal and external audit recommendations
- progress on major capital schemes
- staffing and establishment reports.

As well as considering the above on a monthly basis, there will also be financial information that the board will need to consider every year, notably:

- the annual report and accounts including quality accounts
- financial plans
- the annual audit letter.

The board should also be updated regularly about any new systems and policy initiatives affecting the NHS. The board needs to consider the potential impact of any such developments and prepare for their implementation as well as identify and evaluate any potential risks.

Information produced for both internal and external purposes should be derived from the same financial system so as to ensure that decisions throughout the organisation are made on a consistent basis.

Chapter 12: Treasury and Cash Flow Management

12.1 Introduction

One area where FTs differ from NHS trusts is that they have 'the freedom to invest money for the purposes of, or in connection with, their functions'.[46] However, they are responsible for ensuring that full account is taken of any risks and best practice – Monitor has issued guidance both for managing operating cash and in relation to major investments.

12.2 What is Treasury Management?

Monitor's guidance – Managing Operating Cash in NHS Foundation Trusts – refers to treasury management as being 'the set of policies, strategies and transactions that a company adopts and implements to manage its cash resources, to raise finance at acceptable cost and risk, and to reduce interest rate, foreign exchange and commodity price risks as well as in the conduct of its relationships with its financial stakeholders (mainly banks)'.

A similar definition is used by the Chartered Institute of Public Finance and Accountancy (CIPFA) in its Code of Practice – 'the management of the organisation's cash flows, its banking, money market and capital market transactions; the effective control of the risks associated with those activities; and the pursuit of optimum performance consistent with those risks'.[47]

In relation to treasury management, the key point to bear in mind is that FTs are dealing with public money and they must ensure that they invest it wisely and safely. Monitor has issued guidance in relation to both short and long term investments to help ensure that this is the case.

12.3 Operating Cash Management

Operating cash management refers to the investment of surplus cash that needs to be available within 12 months to support an FT's day-to-day activities and must therefore be both safe and easily available that is, liquid. Monitor's guidance in this area emphasises that the aims of an FT should be to:

- 'ensure a competitive return on surplus cash, with an acceptable risk profile
- manage the financial risk associated with operational activities such as interest rate and foreign currency risks
- ensure availability of competitively priced funding for working capital with an acceptable risk profile'.[48]

---

[46] Risk Evaluation for Investment Decisions by NHS Foundation Trusts, Monitor, 2009: www.monitor-nhsft.gov.uk/home/our-publications/browse-category/guidance-foundation-trusts/mandatory-guidance/risk-evaluation-
[47] Treasury Management in the Public Services: Code of Practice and Cross-Sectoral Guidance Notes, 2011, CIPFA, – www.cipfa.org.uk
[48] Managing Operating Cash in NHS Foundation Trusts, Monitor, 2009: www.monitor-nhsft.gov.uk/sites/default/files/publications/Managing_cash_final.pdf

Although Monitor's guidance is not mandatory it 'strongly encourages' FTs to invest any surplus operating cash in 'safe harbour investments' and to have a written cash management policy.

Safe harbour investments

Safe harbour investments are those investments that have a low risk and high liquidity such as money market deposits, government and local authority bonds, certificates of deposit and sterling commercial paper. Monitor's guidance[49] sets out the criteria that an investment must meet to be classed as 'safe harbour'. These are that the investment must:

- meet permitted rating requirements issued by a recognised rating agency
- be held at a permitted institution
- have a defined maximum maturity date of 3 months
- be denominated in sterling
- pay interest at a fixed, floating, or discount rate
- be within the preferred 'concentration limit'.

The 'concentration limit' seeks to safeguard an FT's investments by not having them concentrated with one institution subject to a threshold amount- spreading investments between institutions minimises the risk to the FT. See Monitor's guidance for more on each criterion. It should be noted that safe harbor investments are treated as cash balances for the purpose of calculating the liquidity ratio.

Monitor does not expect FTs to invest surplus operating cash outside of safe harbour investments. To the extent that an FT does so, it should only be for the management of operational risk (foreign exchange risk or interest rate risk for example) and never for speculative purposes. Any *non* safe harbour investments should be reported as exceptions in line with Monitor's Compliance Framework – they will be excluded from the cash balances included in the liquidity rating (see section 5.3) and their impact on the FT's overall financial risk rating will be considered.

Cash management policy

According to Monitor's guidance, a cash management policy should cover:

- objectives – for each main area for example, cash forecasting and investment of surplus cash. An objective in relation to investing surplus cash is typically to obtain a competitive return within defined risk limits
- attitude to risk – for each of the areas identified in 'objectives' for example, risk profile of investments and institutions might be defined by the safe harbour provisions
- organisation and responsibilities – Monitor 'strongly recommends' that an investment committee is set up, chaired by a non-executive director. The responsibilities of the board of directors, finance director and treasury/accounts function are also covered here

---

[49] Managing Operating Cash in NHS Foundation Trusts, Monitor, 2009:
www.monitor-nhsft.gov.uk/sites/default/files/publications/Managing_cash_final.pdf

- bank relationships and cash management – to set out relationships with key banks and the services they provide such as deposit taking, working capital facilities, bank accounts, and cash management
- reporting – reports that will be produced (daily/weekly/monthly) and their circulation for example, reports on market movements, analysis of investments (performance, liquidity and security) and bank relationships
- performance management – how performance will be measured and monitored for example, against the three month London Interbank Bid Rate (LIBID)
- controls – how the FT will ensure treasury activities are operating as they should.

Monitor's guide gives more details and includes an anonymised example of a private sector cash management policy.

As with all organisations it is important to manage cash effectively. For FTs this is vital. In particular, FTs should have a good cash management policy and a strong credit control department that reports aged receivables (debtors) to the board of directors. Inventory (stock) control is also important and should be managed – poor control leads to higher levels of inventory than necessary and potentially insufficient cash to pay payables (creditors). Poor management of receivables or inventory will result in less than optimum levels of income being generated from short term investments.

12.4 Medium and Long Term Investments

As well as having greater freedom in relation to the way they manage operating cash on a short term basis, FTs also have more scope than other NHS trusts when it comes to medium to long term investments such as major capital items, mergers and joint ventures. However, when considering these 'high risk' investments FTs must follow guidance set down by Monitor in Risk Evaluation for Investment Decisions by NHS Foundation Trusts. This guidance defines 'high risk' investments and sets out best practice principles. In particular, Monitor recommends that FTs:

- develop a written investment policy which covers:
  - the investment committee's functions and structure
  - the FT's investment philosophy and objectives
  - the attitude to risk and process for risk management
  - decision rights (roles, responsibilities and approval limits)
  - the process for evaluating and managing investments
- establish an investment committee – although they are not mandatory they are strongly recommended by Monitor as best practice for managing operating cash purposes and 'if major investment is being proposed' (see section 4.7)
- confirm that the FT has the legal power to make the proposed investment
- engage experienced independent external advisers early on to advise on proposed transactions
- use a 'thorough evaluation, execution and monitoring process' to evaluate proposed investments.

More detail is set out in Monitor's guide, available under the publications section of its website.

In the context of an FT's approach to investments, it is important to note that Monitor's Compliance Framework requires them to report any proposed major investments or divestments if certain criteria are met for example, if the income attributable to a contract with a non-healthcare organisation is greater than 5% of the FT's income. Monitor 'does not have any role in approving such plans unless the trust is being escalated or is in significant breach, but it will consider their impact on the NHS foundation trust's risk ratings and communicate this to trust boards'.[50] See section 5.3 for more about Monitor's Compliance Framework and risk ratings.

12.5 Business Cases

Another important element in an FT's overall investment strategy is an effective approach to the development and use of business cases. A business case is a planning and management tool that helps ensure that any proposed investments:

- are supported by a robust case for change
- optimise value for money
- are commercially viable
- are financially affordable
- are achievable.

For FTs it is particularly important that a business case clearly identifies where and how income will be generated. Sensitivity analysis and risk play an important part in any business case and an exit strategy should also be developed in case any income (or other) assumptions prove to be inaccurate. The HFMA has published detailed guidance on business cases if you want to know more.[51]

Unlike NHS trusts, FTs do not have delegated limits in relation to business cases. However they should make reference to Monitor's Compliance Framework and specifically the sections on major investments and disinvestments as to the circumstances under which they will be required to obtain the approval of the regulator before they proceed with their proposals.

12.6 Working Capital Facilities

What is a working capital facility?

Working capital is the money and assets that an organisation can call upon to finance its day-to-day operations – for example, paying wages, overheads and buying inventory – that produce the goods or services supplied to customers.

Working capital facilities are made available by banks to their customers to help smooth out any volatility in cash flow resulting from the different timing and frequencies of their income and outgoings. For example, if an FT is waiting for contract income and does not currently

---

[50] Compliance Framework, Monitor, 2011/12: www.monitor-nhsft.gov.uk
[51] Public Sector Business Cases using the Five Case Model: a toolkit, HFMA, 2007 – www.hfma.org.uk

have the cash in the bank to pay bills that are due, it can draw down from its working capital facility to bridge the gap.

Why do foundation trusts need to have a working capital facility?

NHS trusts can manage cash shortages by drawing down a working capital loan from the Department. This arrangement requires SHA support as they provide the assurance role. The assessment of loan applications by the Department will take into account the cash available and the prudential borrowing limit of the trust concerned. However FTs do not have this option and need to make their own arrangements for covering any cash shortages that might arise.

Securing a working capital facility is prudent business practice, providing an 'insurance policy' for cash flow and improving liquidity. However for the majority of FTs, it is effectively a requirement as it contributes to the overall financial risk rating awarded by Monitor. The overall rating is important as it reflects the underlying financial health of the FT and influences both the amount of long term borrowing an FT can enter into and the frequency and intensity of monitoring by the regulator.

Chapter 13: Direct Taxation

13.1 Introduction

The April 2004 Budget included an announcement that commercial activities of foundation trusts would be brought within the scope of corporation tax. This initiative was intended to 'level the playing field' between the public and private sectors. However, other factors such as differences in pension contribution funding, post graduate training contributions and the application of value added tax (VAT) would also need to be addressed to produce a genuinely level playing field with the private healthcare sector. These issues and the application of corporation tax in the private sector are not covered here.

There was some concern following this announcement as to what constituted a 'commercial activity' and how taxable profits on such activities would be calculated without incurring significant overhead costs. As a result, the introduction was deferred until Her Majesty's Revenue and Customs (HMRC) and the Department could produce suitable guidance for FTs to explain how the measures would be applied in practice. This guidance was issued in September 2005.[52] However, inconsistency between FTs and other NHS trusts remains – although it is moderated to a degree by the inclusion of de minimis limits (a lower limit below which no action is required).

To that end, and following extensive debate and consultation, the Treasury announced in October 2009 that the decision had been taken to defer the planned implementation of the legislation. This was to allow further consideration in relation to the introduction of the arrangements, the definitions to be used and how they would be applied to all public healthcare providers, with the subsequent intention to apply corporation tax for all healthcare providers from April 2011. During the run-up to the May 2010 general election, the application of corporation tax was put on further hold and no further consultation has since taken place, nor has any revised guidance been issued by the Department or HMRC.

The following sections therefore are based on the guidance received in 2005, updated to incorporate the latest corporation tax rates which are subject to change by future legislation.

13.2 Are Activities Taxable?

The guidance aims to make the assessment of whether an activity is taxable a mechanical one – and a flowchart is provided below for this purpose:

---

[52] Guidance on the Tax Treatment of Non-core Healthcare Activities of NHS Foundation Trusts, HMRC: www.hmrc.gov.uk

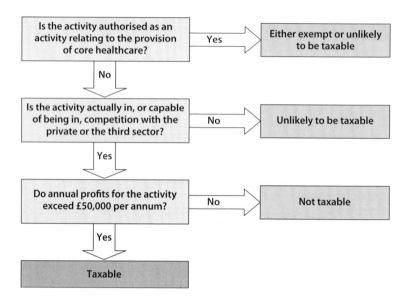

Step 1: Is the activity authorised as an activity relating to the provision of core healthcare?

Although originally thought not to be taxable, many healthcare services are subject to a tendering process, where NHS hospitals may be competing with the independent or third sectors. The current guidance indicates that 'any activity authorised by Monitor under section 14(1) of the Health and Social Care (Community Health and Standard) Act 2003, will not be treated as a commercial activity for corporation tax purposes'. Therefore all NHS funded patient treatment income is likely to be exempt from a charge and privately funded healthcare is also unlikely to be taxable.

Step 2: Is the activity actually in or capable of being in, competition with the private or third sector?

The second step is to consider whether the activity is in competition (or is capable of being in competition) with the private or third sector. The main factor for an activity to be (potentially) exempt at this stage is if it is 'ancillary to core healthcare provision' and therefore focused 'inwardly' (that is, for the benefit of patients, staff and visitors). Examples of such activities are given below:

- likely to be exempt:
  - staff canteens
  - car parking
  - interest receivable
- likely to be taxable:
  - exploitation of intellectual property
  - commercial laundry
  - selling services to other organisations

○ sale of consultancy services
○ commercial manufacture and sale of drugs.

The key phrase here is 'likely to be'. The current guidance indicates that where an FT is in doubt as to whether an income stream is deemed to be commercial advice should be sought from HMRC who will then determine whether a Treasury Order to tax is put in place. Failure to advise HMRC of a potential commercial activity that exceeds the de-minimus limit (see below) may result in interest and penalty charges being recovered by HMRC in addition to the unpaid tax.

Step 3: Do the profits for the activity exceed the de minimis limit?

When determining whether or not an activity is subject to corporation tax and given it has passed the first two tests, the third step is to decide whether it is above the de minimis limit (£50,000 profit per activity). Therefore any activity that is not excluded from each of these steps where the profits exceed £50,000 will fall to be taxable. The application of this limit aims to ensure that '...relatively small transaction streams, which might in themselves constitute a trading activity, are not brought into the scope of tax, thereby preventing unnecessary administrative burdens'.[53]

13.3 Trading Subsidiary Companies

Although the mitigation of corporation taxation is not covered in the 2005 guidance, one potential solution is for those FTs operating taxable activities to set up a trading subsidiary company. The trading activities may then be operated through the company, which will be fully liable to corporation tax. The company could then 'gift aid' its profits to the charitable funds of the FT, reducing the tax liability to zero. An additional benefit of this approach would be the ability of the charity to purchase medical equipment exempt from VAT.

The guidance encourages FTs to operate subsidiary companies where activities are likely to be significant. There are some additional costs (and risks) associated with this approach, and it is possible that the approach could be deemed to be avoidance of the tax liability. Finance directors of FTs requiring advice on setting up a company to carry on commercial non-core healthcare activities should consult professional advisers. They may also contact their HMRC office for advice on the associated corporation tax issues.

13.4 Calculating the Profits of a Trade

The profits of non-core healthcare activities carried out by FTs, including capital allowances[54] if applicable, should be calculated in the same way as for any other trader. However, there are some factors which may be particularly relevant when calculating the profits of a trade.

---

[53] Guidance on the Tax Treatment of Non-core Healthcare Activities of NHS Foundation Trusts, HMRC: www.hmrc.gov.uk
[54] Ordinarily depreciation and amortisation charges on capitalised assets are not allowable deductible expenses for the purpose of calculating taxable profits. Instead entities will deduct a capital allowance from their taxable profit calculations. Capital allowances are calculated by applying 'Writing Down Allowances (WDAs)' on an annual basis.

As well as deducting direct expenditure of the trade, the FT should also deduct indirect expenditure that it has incurred and which is attributable to the trade. For example, if the trade is carried on in the trust's premises it will normally be proper to allocate a proportion of the associated premise costs to the trade such as:

- heat and light
- rent
- building repairs and maintenance.

Other indirect costs which may be partly attributable to the trade are:

- indirect employee costs
- computer costs
- telephone charges
- postage costs
- accountancy and legal fees
- general administration.

The proper basis to be used when apportioning indirect costs will depend on the activity in question. In the case of the use of premises, the apportionment might be based on the floor area allocated to the trade. In the case of indirect employee costs, the apportionment might be based on the amount of time specifically devoted to the trade as compared with other activities.

13.5 Calculation and Payment of Corporation Tax Liability

The calculation of the corporation tax due on the profits from a trading activity can be seen in the table below:

	£	£
Trading income:		
Adjusted profit	X	
Less: capital allowances	X	
Tax adjusted trading profit		X
Less: donations to charity (gift aid)		X
Profits chargeable to corporation tax (PCTCT)		X

The corporation tax rates for 2011/12 are:

Small profits rate   20% (if profits are below £300,000)

Main rate   26% (if profits are above £1.5m)

Profits between £300,000 and £1.5m are taxed at a marginal rate of 27.5%. In the first budget of the coalition government on 22 June 2010, the main rate of corporation tax for 2011/12 was reduced by 1% to 27%, with further annual reductions of 1% for the following three years, until it reaches 23% in 2014/15.

Further guidance is awaited from HMRC and the Department as to when corporation tax will be applied to the NHS but as noted in section 13.1 if corporation tax is applied to the NHS, the earliest it is likely to be effective is for the financial year 2012/13. In this case the first set of accounts to be affected will be for the year ending 31 March 2013 with the first payment of tax due on 1 January 2014 and the first corporation tax return due by April 2013.

Further guidance can be found via the HMRC's web site at www.hmrc.gov.uk.

Chapter 14: Insurance

14.1 Scope

Prior to the introduction of FTs NHS bodies were expressly forbidden from taking out commercial insurance, except in the following specific circumstances:

- motor insurance – on the grounds that an efficient commercial market already existed
- income generation
- PFI developments.

NHS bodies were free to choose to obtain cover via the NHSLA[55] through the Risk Pooling Scheme for Trusts (RPST) which was an 'unfunded' scheme. An unfunded scheme only charges premiums based on current claims and claims likely to occur in the next 12 months. This approach makes the scheme contributions cheaper than premiums for comparable commercial insurance cover, particularly in the earlier years.

The schemes provided by the NHSLA do not provide the full range of cover that an organisation operating in a truly 'commercial' environment would require (see below). While remaining eligible for membership of the RPST, FTs are beyond the explicit direction of the Secretary of State for Health and so can choose to take out additional or alternative commercial insurance if required. Indeed, since FTs have a duty to remain a going concern, many boards have taken the view that additional commercial insurance is essential.

The RPST is subdivided into two separate schemes, the Property Expenses Scheme (PES) and the Liability to Third Party Scheme (LTPS) and we'll look at each in turn. It is worth noting that there is no flexibility in relation to excesses or the extent of the cover.

14.2 Property Expenses Scheme (PES)

The PES covers all buildings and equipment owned by or the responsibility of the member trust. Cover is subject to a 'deductible' of £20,000 for each and every buildings claim and one of £20,000 in relation to each contents claim. There is an 'upper limit' for each organisation of £1m for each incident. There are three main categories of cover – property damage, business interruption and contract works, each having a £1m limit. Therefore a total claim could be up to £3m (less applicable deductibles).

This upper limit allows for strategic decision making in the event of a catastrophic incident which could allow for the relocation of services rather than a straightforward re-provision of what was lost.

PES also covers engineering risks (but not statutory inspection) with a limit of £1m; fidelity guarantee, with a limit of £250,000; money (limits for cash are below the scheme excess) and goods in transit (limit equates to scheme deductible).

---

[55] NHSLA web site: www.nhsla.com/home.htm

Many FTs have chosen therefore to obtain commercial 'top-up' cover – in effect, property cover with an excess of £1m. This commercial cover can be obtained to extend the scope of the cover provided by the NHSLA policies as follows:

- loss of income – the NHSLA business interruption cover does not include any loss of NHS income. The cover that is provided (increased cost of working and loss of profit from income generation activities) can be topped up
- terrorism – the NHSLA policy includes terrorism cover up to the scheme limit. Additional cover is available as an 'add on'
- fidelity guarantee – the cover provided by the NHSLA scheme for money embezzled/ stolen by employees is limited to £250,000. Monitor's liquidity requirements mean that most FTs routinely hold and invest cash balances far in excess of this limit and additional cover should be considered
- contract works – where Joint Name Contract Conditions apply to contracted works complications may arise as the PES does not allow a third party to be named. Responsibility to insure can be passed to the contractor (at a cost), but often it is less risky for the FT to arrange additional insurance. In addition, joint names cover is not available under PES for existing structures. When works are being undertaken on existing structures it is often the case that the FT, as employer, is responsible for insuring the existing structures in joint names. If commercial top up cover is in place, an 'extension in cover' can be sought from the insurer for claims above the excess. However the contractor should be made to retain responsibility for damage he causes up to the level of the excess
- engineering risks – top up to the £1m provided by PES
- money
- goods in transit.

14.3 Liability to Third Party Scheme (LTPS)

The NHSLA LTPS provides unlimited cover subject to the applicable excesses, for:

- employers' liability
- public and products liability (NHS, income generation activities within the NHS and specified income generation activities outside of the NHS)
- directors' and officers' liability
- professional indemnity (NHS, income generation activities within the NHS and specified income generation activities outside of the NHS).

It is worth noting that limits apply to pollution liability (£10m per year) and financial loss (£250,000 per year). Personal accident cover is provided to employees on an emergency call out or patient transfer or to staff who are assaulted while at work with a maximum payable per incident of £250,000.

FTs therefore often obtain additional cover in the following areas:

- public and products liability and where applicable, non clinical professional indemnity cover for non-NHS income generation activities

- directors and officers – to cover activities that fall outside of the 'Trust Relevant Function' for example, private contracts
- personal accident – some NHS activities have been targeted and the benefits payable increased for example, crash teams and blue light transfers
- travel cover
- clinical trials – commercial insurance can be sought for clinical trials when indemnities are not available from the manufacturer.

It is worth remembering that FTs should consult the NHSLA and their own insurance brokers to receive specific advice when considering insurance requirements.

The HFMA has produced a briefing in relation to insurance for foundation trusts which can be found via the website www.hfma.org.uk.